Self-Neglecting Elders

Self-Neglecting Elders
A CLINICAL DILEMMA

EDITED BY

Eloise Rathbone-McCuan
&
Dorothy R. Fabian

Foreword by
Richard L. Schiefelbusch

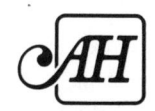

AUBURN HOUSE
New York • Westport, Connecticut • London

Library of Congress Cataloging-in-Publication Data

Self-neglecting elders : a clinical dilemma / edited by Eloise Rathbone-
    McCuan and Dorothy R. Fabian ; foreword by Richard L.
    Schiefelbusch.
        p.   cm.
    Includes bibliographical references and index.
    ISBN 0-86569-047-2 (alk. paper)
    1. Aged—Health and hygiene. 2. Aged—Mental health. 3. Self-
care, Health. 4. Geriatric psychiatry. I. Rathbone-McCuan,
Eloise. II. Fabian, Dorothy R., 1923–
RA564.8.S463 1992
613'.0438—dc20   91-36343

British Library Cataloguing in Publication Data is available.

Copyright © 1992 by Eloise Rathbone-McCuan and Dorothy R. Fabian

All rights reserved. No portion of this book may be
reproduced, by any process or technique, without the
express written consent of the publisher.

Library of Congress Catalog Card Number: 91-36343
ISBN 0-86569-047-2

First published in 1992

Auburn House, 88 Post Road West, Westport, CT 06881
An imprint of Greenwood Publishing Group, Inc.

Printed in the United States of America

The paper used in this book complies with the
Permanent Paper Standard issued by the National
Information Standards Organization (Z39.48–1984).

10   9   8   7   6   5   4   3   2   1

I dedicate this book in memory of my friend and colleague Dr. Philip Weiler who died in June 1991 as this work was being completed for publication. He made many pioneering advances in the field of gerontology and I was fortunate to share part of that adventurous journey for many years. First colleague, best colleague — I will keep our faith as I continue the work we began so long ago. You and those who provide adult protective services and case management supports to elderly clients attempting to sustain their independence have made an important difference in this world.

L.R.M.

To my husband, Maine Channeling, and the patients and staff of the Geriatric Hip Fracture Program at the Hospital for Joint Diseases Orthopaedic Institute.

D.R.F.

Contents

Foreword by Richard L. Schiefelbusch   ix
Preface   xi

I OVERVIEW

1   Elder Self-Neglect: A Blurred Concept   3
     Dorothy R. Fabian and Eloise Rathbone-McCuan

2   A General Framework for Elder Self-Neglect   13
     Eloise Rathbone-McCuan and Mary Bricker-Jenkins

II SYSTEMS CONSIDERATIONS

3   Ethical Issues in Working with Self-Neglect   27
     Stephen J. Cutler and William A. Tisdale

4   Psychiatric and Biomedical Considerations in Self-Neglect   46
     Raymond Vickers

5   A Family Systems Perspective of Self-Neglect   71
     Caroline T. Wilner and Nancy R. Vosler

III SPECIAL RISKS AND SUBGROUPS

6 Institutional Care Settings and Self-Neglect   91
Joan K. Hashimi and Linda Withers

7 Older Developmentally Disabled Adults and Self-Neglect   107
Allene M. Jackson and Cynthia Compton

8 Geriatric Alcoholism and Self-Neglect   127
Larry Dyer

9 Geriatric Protective Services and Self-Neglect   144
Eloise Rathbone-McCuan and Marilyn C. Whalen

10 Conclusion: Research and Clinical Directions in Self-Neglect   161
Eloise Rathbone-McCuan and Dorothy R. Fabian

Bibliography   173
Index   187
About the Contributors   195

Foreword

Richard L. Schiefelbusch

The number of self-neglecting elders seems to be increasing. However, various cultures, through ages past, have reported hermits and "sack cloth and ashes" members who expired amid evidence of poverty and squalor even though family or authorities eventually found wealth in various containers on their living premises. From a more general perspective, it might be concluded that benign self-neglect is at least a possible accompaniment of aging and in some instances becomes a tragic indicator of social deterioration during the latter stages of the life cycle.

More often self-neglect seems to be manifest in the elder's lack of effort or aptitude for self-advocacy and, thus, presents the appearance of isolation or apathy that accompanies societal neglect. These and other possibilities are documented and discussed in this book.

As stated in the book's title, the phenomenon of self-neglect produces a dilemma for caregivers and family members who wish to support the aging member and to accept his or her preferred lifestyle as far as possible. It is not easy to ask other adults to upscale their lifestyles. Likewise, it is not comfortable to direct or otherwise induce change leading to altered preferences. The dilemma may be intensified by individualized deviances in a client's behavior.

Approaches to social/behavioral treatment in care facilities virtually require the caregiver to include the client's preferences in regard to goals, daily activities, and modes of living. However, if these preferences are seen as self-destructive or denegating, the therapist is placed in an awkward ethical or strategic position, especially if the client has been encouraged to maintain autonomy in the selection of personal goals and activity preferences. If an aging individual has been allowed to make personal choices and to assume the consequences for those choices, the caregiver cannot very well restrict or counter those choices on a daily basis.

Apparently, the authors of *Self-Neglecting Elders* have exposed a strategic problem that requires further analysis and additional client/caregiver approaches of negotiation. One suspects, naturally, that tendencies leading to self-neglect spring from individual pathologies of various kinds that reduce health, energies, and personal pride. If so, perhaps the primary conditions can be treated and the self-neglect thereby reduced. If indeed it works that way, the problem is a second-order effect. However, to assume a direct causal relationship may be premature. For instance, we would be leaving out changes in self-esteem that may stem from declining favorable feedback and/or altering social motivations. In any event, self-neglect is a condition that must be reckoned with, and its place in the life patterns of aging groups must be analyzed in strategic detail.

This book suggests a wide range of research activity and points toward further directions to plan it such research. A logical initial objective for such research is to understand the distribution of self-neglect in the elder population and the factors that influence its distribution. Before that objective is reached, we may be impelled to confront the ubiquitous conditions of aged persons who ignore some aspect of their self-care that may create some risk and those in a serious state of self-neglect resulting in physical, mental, or combined impairments. Those distinctions require sensitive analysis and careful monitoring — in short, the compassionate side of caregiving.

Preface

Necessity, the sister of invention, leads all of us down strange and unpredictable pathways. Community outreach through comprehensive case management services and case work follow-up in adult protective services were identifying a growing number of elder self-neglect cases. Staff were troubled by the complex ambiguity and severity of these situations and requested direction from us as accessible consultants for team case reviews. Most of the available literature proved to be somewhat limited to medical and nursing perspectives. Publications were available on elder-abuse, not our focus, and the term "elder-neglect" related to caregiver behaviors. Contacts with academic peers often resulted in a half apology that they were not familiar with the term. A few suggested we contact practitioners they knew and described as people "in the frontlines of practice" and "surviving in the practice trenches."

We began sending letters and making phone calls to those suggested and to others we had worked with. The range of reactions we received was somewhat foreboding. An experienced urban geriatric psychotherapist said, "Well, I don't have contact with homeless elderly, so what would I know?" A rural public health nurse responded by saying, "Yes, I have attempted a few unsuccessful home visits and could never get inside to talk to the people." A social worker said, "Well, self-neglect is an oxymoron if I've ever heard one. What are you talking about?"

Some of our contacts discussed their ideas about self-neglect and sent us brief case studies. One letter, now laughed about as our predestination, included the statement, "I continue to be horrified by the conditions of isolation and poverty facing some of my clients, and I am confused by other elderly people who live in the worst neglect, but, in fact, they could pay my salary for a lifetime. Why don't you try writing a book on elder self-neglect as a clinical dilemma?" Shortly thereafter, over the crackling phone lines in a New England blizzard, we decided this book should be written, to pull together what sparse accounts do exist with what our authors know about elder self-neglect from their own professional experiences and perspective. After all, knowledge building often begins with subjective reality that flows into and greatly enhances the objective domain.

The reader may wonder why we did not begin with one comprehensive definition of elder self-neglect, thereby providing a more structured conceptual framework from which to organize the material. We were not willing to address this complex and vague issue by superimposing a single definition onto authors who came from very different perspectives on elder self-neglect.

Future efforts should emerge from a more solid research base than is now available. Many of the questions appropriate for scientific investigation are raised in this work. Until and after multidisciplinary research begins, the "practice wisdom" contributed in this collection will be an important reference point to guide empirical work and clinical program design.

The book opens with the historical background of ancient to current community and professional responses to self-neglecting elders. These responses include offensive characterizations and euphemistic clinical descriptions of the problem. The second chapter provides a general framework that describes the processes involved in elder self-neglect; that is, how does an elderly person reach the point where self-neglect threatens the life-sustaining desire for independence that may change into one of the greatest sources of risk to personal autonomy. The middle section of this book addresses problems that have systems implications encompassing the broad phenomenon of elder self-neglect: the ethical issues that confront society as a whole and have specific implications for clinical practice, biopsychological factors that are central to client assessment and subsequent therapeutic interventions, and family systems considerations that may come into play to cause and/or eliminate elder self-neglect.

Selected subgroups of aging persons known to have special self-neglect risks are given attention in the final section of the book. Nursing home residents, often thought to be monitored and protected against risks, have the potentiality for serious self-neglect. Problems of and solutions to self-neglect among older developmentally disabled persons emerging into independent living experiences give a new perspective on community programming applicable to reducing self-neglect problems. Alcoholism, a multidimensional problem that potentially grows more severe with age, is described in relation to its association with elder self-neglect. Self-neglect cases served by adult protective service programs and the structure of these programs are considered at local, state, and national levels. The concluding chapter discusses areas of research and knowledge building likely to advance greater understanding of elder self-neglect.

Sincere appreciation is extended to the administrators and staff of the Colmery-O'Neil V.A. Medical Center in Topeka, Kansas, who provided many resources necessary to bring this project to its conclusion. Numerous boxes of red pens and years of encouragement were supplied by Terry Harbert. Judith Wartman, Susan Tebb, Nancy Intermill, Karen Cook, and Linda Halleck all helped to resolve problems and supported the project at some critical points. Chuck Bland is thanked many times for his assistance.

Our hope, as editors and authors, is that this pioneering effort will provide a departure point for the ultimate destination — further scientific and clinical investigation as well as expanded and adequately financed health and social services.

I

OVERVIEW

1

Elder Self-Neglect: A Blurred Concept

Dorothy R. Fabian and Eloise Rathbone-McCuan

Self-neglect has been emerging poignantly as one of the many troublesome problems that beset the elderly. It is a source of anxiety and frustration for practitioners, family members, and the community because self-neglecting elders may present themselves in antisocial and life-threatening situations. That is because self-neglect is frequently manifest by disregard of the needs of both the self and the environment. Usually, self-neglect results from physical and/or mental impairments that reduce the elder's ability to perform essential life tasks. There may be no shame about the situation, and outside help may be refused or passively sabotaged.

Self-neglect is multifaceted and seems to be at once situational, behavioral, and attitudinal. It may include insufficient self-awareness, wayward self-definition, and inadequate self-prioritization. There are social, physical, emotional, and economic factors to be understood, all of which, in varying combinations, can produce self-neglect. It may be referred to as a symptom often associated with depression, as both a physical and an environmental condition resulting from poverty, and as a behavioral characteristic emerging from mental incompetence. It is fraught with conceptual complexity and ethical ambiguity. In addition, widespread confusion about the causes and treatment of self-neglect may lead to its being dealt with intuitively.

Without a conceptual framework or an adequate knowledge base about elder self-neglect, it is not difficult to understand why inconsistent, incomplete, and incorrect measures are taken to deal with all the human needs and problems faced by aged clients. There is little agreement about the clinical work necessary and appropriate to ameliorate self-neglect.

Our exploration of self-neglect began in 1985 while working on clinical assessment and case management services for high-risk elders residing in the community. We realized that many of the elderly who could most benefit from services and care provided by social, medical, and psychiatric practitioners were being described as neglected, by themselves or by others. The research on elder abuse was increasing, but little attention was directed to self-neglect as a condition often observed in isolated elderly. A clinical framework for providing services to isolated elders had been developed (Rathbone-McCuan and Hashimi, 1982), but the disregard of self-neglect was a clinical impediment. As a result, this book is a collaborative effort among authors and editors to advance clinical work with elderly clients who are thought to be neglecting their needs and placing themselves at high risk of further and devastating deterioration. Through the contributed papers we have attempted to unravel the complexities of elder self-neglect and to identify, describe, and address the situational, behavioral, and attitudinal qualities associated with self-neglect in the geriatric population.

SELF-NEGLECT IN THE LITERATURE

Self-neglect is probably not a new phenomenon. Isolated, frequently unkempt, and often eccentric individuals such as hermits, witches, tramps, and recluses have long been depicted in the social history, literature, folklore, and opera of Western society. These were the early sources of cultural stereotypes depicting extreme examples of self-neglecters. Often arousing fear, discomfort, and disgust, some of these men and women were seen as mentally ill; some were expected to be able to call on fearful supernatural powers; some were thought to hoard treasure. All were considered strange and lived on the social, if not the physical, periphery of their communities. The local populace tended to subject such individuals to jeers, taunts, beatings, and ostracism. Imprisonment, banishment, or violent death at times followed attention by authorities.

The stereotyping of elderly self-neglecters continues through mass media efforts to keep the U.S. homeless population visible as a newsworthy phenomenon. An increasing amount of contemporary medical and psychiatric literature has addressed gross neglect as a manifestation of individual dysfunction even though it is not clear that the rate and severity of self-neglect in the aging population have increased. Clinical case studies and reports of small samples attempt to verify that self-neglecters become embroiled with the police, wander into emergency rooms, and plague social service agencies. Lurid published accounts lead the public to conclude that high-cost care to improve the condition of these persons provides no long-term benefits and that many of those who do receive community resources will eventually die in very deteriorated conditions.

In attempts to understand self-neglect, certain observers noted an age-related dimension. Macmillan and Shaw (1966) used the senile breakdown syndrome to describe persons failing to maintain levels of cleanliness that the community found acceptable:

> The usual picture is that of an old woman living alone, though men and married couples suffering from the condition are also found. She, her garments, her possessions, and her house are filthy. She may be verminous and there may be feces and pools of urine on the floor. These people are often tolerated for years by the neighbors, who may suddenly decide that they cannot stand this state of affairs any longer and report the case to various organizations, such as the police or the health department (p. 1032).

Clark, Mankikar, and Gray (1975), referring to the fourth-century Greek philosopher Diogenes, who reportedly admired lack of shame, outspokenness, and contempt for social organization, suggested the phrase "Diogenes Syndrome" to characterize elderly patients who appeared filthy and unkempt, whose homes were dirty and untidy and usually full of hoarded rubbish, but who showed no shame for these circumstances. Although not necessarily poor or in substandard housing, these self-neglecting individuals were usually known to social service agencies, whose efforts were frequently resisted.

The term "Diogenes Syndrome" became a stereotype for self-neglecting elders perceived as grossly neglectful of their person and the environment, who displayed not only a lack of shame but also contempt for, or at least disinterest in, the recommendations of neighbors, family members, health providers, or the community at large. The Diogenes Syndrome is used to describe patients in at least one nursing care study (Cornwall, 1981) as well as in a paper on psychotic disturbances (Klosterkotter and Peters, 1985). It is also referred to in a study of the social breakdown syndrome in community-dwelling elderly (Radebaugh, Hooper, and Gruenberg, 1987).

The construct "social breakdown syndrome" (Gruenberg and Zusman, 1964; Gruenberg, Brandon, and Kasius, 1966; Brandon and

Gruenberg, 1966; Gruenberg, 1967; Zusman, 1967; Gruenberg, Snow, and Bennett, 1969; Archer and Gruenberg, 1982; Radebaugh, Hooper, and Gruenberg, 1987) was developed to refer to psychiatric problems unrelated to specific age groups but describing "progressive chronic deterioration chiefly by behavior changes which are observable as modifications of personal and social behavior" (Gruenberg, 1967, p. 1481). This behavior results in the breakdown of relationships between an individual and the environment and is marked by an inability or lack of motivation to meet minimal expectations of self-care or to conform to community standards of behavior. As deterioration progresses, the individual may exhibit "gross negligence of self-care and dangerous or annoying behavior." If hospitalization occurs, it is because the patient is believed to be incapable of caring for self and likely to be dangerous to self or others. Gruenberg (1967) further pointed out that "the course (of social breakdown syndrome) can sometimes be indolently progressive, starting mildly and advancing by small increments over several years to an extreme form of no work, no play, frequent soiling, frequent violence, and consistent resistance to all daily self-care activities" (Gruenberg, 1967, p. 1483).

Kuyper and Bengtson (1973) extend the concept of social breakdown syndrome beyond mental illness and suggest its incorporation into a model of normal aging. They interpret the social breakdown syndrome as a series of events during which "an individual's sense of self, ability to mediate between self and society, and orientation to personal mastery are functions of the kinds of social labeling and valuing experienced in aging" (p. 182). The dependency on social labeling occurs because of the kinds of social reorganization that occur in late life, that is, the role loss, vague norms, probable loss of reference groups, and likely decrease in prestige. These losses deprive the individual of usual sources of feedback about roles, behavior, and value and create a vulnerability to "external sources of self-labeling, many of which communicate a stereotyped negative message of the elderly as useless and obsolete" (p. 182). Kuyper and Bengtson's argument, then, is that aging can assume a pathological flavor because changes in the social environment cause individuals to doubt their social competence, which in turn leads to low self-assessment and a continuing reduction of previously employed coping skills. It can be seen that such a process could lead to self-neglect. What is not clear is what proportion of the elderly population suffers social breakdown and why its occurrence is not universal.

On the one hand, although self-neglect was not reported as a common condition in the literature of the 1960s, Macmillan and Shaw (1966) insist that few practitioners working with the elderly escaped encountering the phenomenon. On the other hand, Roe (1977), writing about patients admitted to a hospital for physical problems characterized as "self-neglect," found only 25 cases so diagnosed during a five-year period.

Conditions observed by Cybulska and Rucinski (1986) echo those described by Macmillan and Shaw (1966) of deteriorated self-presentation and slovenly environment attributed to the person's disregard of the setting:

> Patients' homes are conspicuously filthy and neglected ... a strong stale and often suffocating smell ... half-empty bottles, dirty glasses and dishes with rotting food are scattered around and mixed with dirty clothes, books, faded pictures, and old news papers.... The patient ... when confined to bed lies under a pile of ragged grimy blankets, newspapers, or cardboard. Patients appear as if they never undress, wash, or comb their sometimes infested or matted hair (p. 21).

Cybulska and Rucinski found that most of these self-neglecting individuals resented any efforts to "interfere" with their chosen lifestyle, including advisable medical and psychiatric examination.

During the 1980s, hospital emergency rooms and departments of nursing became increasingly inured to filth of person and clothing and emaciation in the poverty-stricken homeless who were brought in for medical attention, but medical personnel also had to deal with elderly individuals who had places to live and sufficient funds to provide the necessities of life but were obviously self-neglectful though stoutly denying their conditions (O'Rawe, 1982). Although the malnutrition and other self-care problems could be corrected while the patients were in the hospital, only education could be offered at discharge. One of the authors of this chapter (Fabian) was present at several case conferences of a specialty hospital's geriatric hip fracture program where similar conditions were reported. The only reason these patients had permitted themselves to be cleansed and examined was that they had fallen and fractured a hip. During follow-up in the community, it was clear that the habitual self-neglectful way of life was resumed and would continue.

One conclusion to be drawn from clinical accounts is that such patients are among the "resistant undesirables" who bother the community because they deviate from some norm of self-maintenance and are not readily inclined to alter their patterns even if they have the economic, physical, and/or cognitive capacity to do so. Neither do they welcome assistance, nor are they likely to follow practitioner recommendations.

CONCEPTUAL AMBIGUITIES

Self-neglect as a clinical concept lacks clarity. When applied, it may produce diagnostic confusion; its etiology is uncertain; and intervention strategies likely to improve the patient's situation are unclear. Although psychiatric functioning may sometimes play a role in the development of self-neglecting behaviors, efforts to describe a syndrome imply that a larger array of behaviors is present, often without clear symptoms of mental illness. Cultural background and lifestyle may play a role, but they are not in themselves causes. Helplessness and increased frailty with aging may have significance but offer little to establish causation. Many older people are not self-neglectful, and many people with disabilities seek out assistance or willingly accept it to help themselves maintain adequate living standards. Alzheimer's disease or related dementias are sometimes characterized by these behaviors in the middle stages of the disease, but many individuals without the diagnosis of a dementia or related cognitive impairments engage in self-neglect that warrants legitimate clinical concern.

Insights into how to treat or resolve self-neglect among the elderly are subject to as much ambiguity as are the diverse explanations of causality. Cybulska and Rucinski (1986) comment:

> Regrettably, when one is faced with a clinical decision whether to intervene or not, the scanty research, medical textbooks, and professional training offer little help. If a crisis occurs in the community, it is often difficult to determine whether the neglect was a result of a consciously determined free choice, some deeply rooted unconscious factors, helplessness, or mental or physical illness (p. 25).

This ambiguity and the contradictions that surround the problem of self-neglect among elderly persons result in decisions regarding intervention that may become mired in a morass of ethical dilemmas. The desire to guarantee a client's personal safety is often pitted against that client's right to self-determination. The struggle to provide some responsible intervention may be experienced at several levels. The first is between the practitioner and the would-be client who is not amenable to assistance but is in rapid decline or dangerous circumstances that can be attributed to self-neglect. Also, the practitioner's effort to obtain access to what the client needs may be frustrated because agencies and organizations controlling resources have not responded in accordance with client need. A third issue may involve matters of jurisdiction over a client, the resources needed by the client, or a combination of the two.

Important ethical questions seem to surface at almost every turn when practitioners are attempting to work with self-neglect problems. Debates about lifestyle and judgments made by others do not entitle society to develop a general policy of pitchforking people into institutional tidiness (Roe, 1987). Even the mentally ill have an increasing amount of protection from those who would help out of concern and from others who would act out of a blatant or subtle desire to control behavior that is considered unacceptable by some sector of the community.

The field of aging needs to consider what guidelines are appropriate to direct intervention around matters of elder self-neglect. Part of that process will involve helping clinicians to gain the expertise to engage the self-neglecting elderly in a process that respects client autonomy to make a choice even if that choice is counter to clinical opinion, that engages clients in a process of decision making rather than mere debate over the decision, that helps clients accomplish steps toward health and well-being, and that facilitates the best outcomes of those decisions, once made and implemented.

SELF-NEGLECT AND COMPLIANCE

To add to the conceptual confusion, the boundaries between self-neglect and treatment compliance seem blurred. Definitional distinctions are especially confusing if self-neglect is narrowly defined as an excessive behavior, which may be either commission or omission of an activity that is both prolonged and dangerous to the individual.

Reed and Leonard (1989) point out, "Self-neglect and noncompliance are similar concepts in that both refer to the client's lack of participation in a prescribed or necessary health care regimen" (p. 42). According to Ramsden (1988), "Compliance" means that "the patient follows medical orders and does what the health care practitioner has instructed" (p. 2). Reed and Leonard (1989) stress that while the focus of compliance is a health-care regimen, in considering self-neglect a great deal of attention must be paid to personal and social-environmental factors. Zola (1986) mentions that the rates for noncompliance are quite high, ranging anywhere from 20 percent to over 70 percent in a patient population, and points out that the rates are higher for the elderly, especially if they are less educated, poor, single, widowed, or divorced.

The medical compliance literature gives particular attention to problems among elderly patients who do not follow a prescribed drug regimen according to physician directive, but there is also reference to the lack of proper nutrition and exercise, absence of personal hygiene, and perpetuation of environmental filth. Other behavioral patterns such as alcohol consumption and smoking and their cessation are also of concern in relation to the elderly patient's medical compliance patterns. However, it is sometimes difficult to discern when a behavior is an aspect of lifestyle and when it is self-neglect severe enough to warrant intervention by the medical and social service delivery systems.

Compliance research has followed several causal lines of analysis that are also applied to the issue of self-neglect even though the latter topic has not yet been the focus of in-depth empirical research. One thesis applied to explain the lack of compliance is anchored in the individual patient's personality or efforts to maintain control over medical routines that dominate daily life. In psychiatry, the lack of medication compliance among persons with long-term mental illness is equated to the behavior of a rebellious child. The clinician has the authority and responsibility to provide the patient with access to the life-enhancing resources available in the form of psychotropic medication. This becomes a parallel to parental right and responsibility.

A patient who refuses to follow the guidelines given for taking medication is defined as noncompliant if he or she varies the use of the prescribed drugs. If patients dispose of the medication, possibly having lost or otherwise misplaced the drugs, they are admonished. Medication utilization among psychiatric patients is a highly complex and important problem, and compliance research that focuses on the interpersonal dynamics of the "uncooperative personality" has little utility for changing the behavior or otherwise increasing the safety and welfare of the patient.

Some researchers have expanded their causal hypotheses beyond the dynamics of the individual patient and have begun to consider how treatment approaches may be intimately involved in compliance levels. Zola (1986) suggests, "The problem of noncompliance (may be) generic to the way we currently deal with chronic disease" (p. 72) and that health personnel may themselves contribute to noncompliance.

There has been some investigation of the interactions between the client and the health professional with regard to the conditions that increase or decrease compliance. Kemp (1988) points out that noncompliance arises as an issue only when more than one individual is involved. This subtle point may hold an important clue to understanding compliance as it specifically relates to persons with chronic conditions, for example, the elderly, where there is the likelihood of an ongoing relationship between clinician and patient. If staff feel pessimistic and helpless when treating older people or if staff have different expectations of the helping process than does the elder, noncompliance may be a more comfortable label than lack of treatment efficacy.

Legal and ethical issues of patient autonomy emerge as central to the practitioner-patient relationship as it applies to treatment compliance. The practitioner has numerous ways to try to influence the patient to accept and act on professional recommendations or prescriptions so as to improve a condition or situation. Guccione (1988) points out that increases in knowledge and the sophistication of technologies have been accompanied by gains in practitioner authority but adds that "the assumption that what is clinically desirable and legally permissible is also automatically ethical cannot be justified" (p. 63). Coy (1989) writes, "As long as health care professionals remain focused on compliance as the goal rather than autonomy enhancement, there is a danger that they will consider autonomy infringements, such as exaggeration of information, to be acceptable, especially if it increases compliance, and thereby increases the patient's functional outcome" (p. 56).

Increasingly, legal and statutory limits and professional sanctions are being placed on the practitioner that serve as boundaries of professional power/influence over patient/clients. These not only apply in cases of medical and psychiatric care but also extend ever greater influence on social service agencies to which the self-neglecting elderly are referred. Respect for autonomy and self-determination and the laws and norms that support these as individual rights have become a vital part of the intervention context. Within that context, the professional must provide necessary information for the individual to make an informed decision and then must act in ways to support the client in the decision-making process.

IS THERE A "TYPICAL" CASE OF SELF-NEGLECT?

In the image that comes to mind when health professionals think of self-neglect, both person and environment are consistently and persistently neglected, and help from the community is either refused or passively sabotaged by noncompliant behaviors. The individual shows no shame regarding this situation and does not, therefore, understand the concerns of the community. Usually, no clear-cut psychopathology is apparent that explains the behavior. Finally, the behavior often places the elder in severe and life-threatening risk, if not immediate, then relatively imminent. However, the pure case rarely exists.

Although a situation is sometimes discovered that exemplifies all these characteristics, most cases involve many causes with many possible directions for solutions. Sometimes organic brain impairment is involved. Strong intervention may be required although the individual's rights need to be protected. Additionally, mental illness may be diverting the elder's attention from the lacks of cleanliness and adequate nutrition. Lifestyle plays a part in the situation. Alcohol and drug abuse may also contribute to, or form the central core of, the problem in some cases. Thus, the stereotypic or "typical" case is actually exceptional. In order to understand the nature of the entire phenomenon of elder self-neglect, we must examine all of its possible causal factors and the socio-medico-legal conditions that currently affect its clinical disposition. We need to resist the impulse to accept stereotypic and simplistic solutions to complex and multicausal problems if we are to make an impact on the issue of self-neglect, which has remained so impervious to current intervention approaches.

The following chapter provides a conceptual framework to accomplish this task.

2
A General Framework for Elder Self-Neglect

Eloise Rathbone-McCuan and Mary Bricker-Jenkins

The purpose of this chapter is to provide a general framework for understanding the condition referred to as elder self-neglect. It is a recognized problem among the elderly population and represents, in many cases, a clinical dilemma for geriatric practitioners. The condition results from an individual's difficulty in obtaining, maintaining, and/or managing the necessities of life independently. Necessities include food that meets at least minimum nutritional requirements, clothing and shelter required for personal safety, health care adequate to prevent or treat debilitating mental or physical conditions, income and financial management to handle routine and personal care expenses, and social-emotional support.

THE CONTEXT OF ELDER SELF-NEGLECT

Problems of self-neglect may range from poor grooming (if it is so poor that it results in the aged person becoming isolated from others) to disintegration of the body that promotes disease and disability or even death. Some of the factors that lead to self-neglect may result from individual conditions, such as mental impairment, that make the person unable to handle basic decisions without guidance and directions from others, interpersonal conditions where neither the individual nor caregivers have knowledge about or ability to obtain needed resources, or environmental conditions that make it difficult or impossible for the person to receive the necessary assistance.

Self-neglecting elders frequently experience harmful situations or live in very inadequate circumstances because mental and/or physical impairments have increased and needed resources have not been made available for declining capacity. Alternatively, elders may fear seeking help because they do not want to be a burden to others or to risk losing privacy or independence, become disoriented because of alcohol misuse or from use or misuse of prescribed medications, become unmotivated to care for self or immobilized because of depression or other psychiatric conditions, or be unaware of resources or services that might be available.

Most conditions that contribute to self-neglect are not understood quickly. It is often easier to observe the consequences of self-neglect if a concerned person is around on a regular basis to understand the daily behavior of the elder at risk. Sometimes an observer's assessment of problems and needs is based on individual perceptions. When professional assessment indicates no risk to the impaired elder, the right to live as he or she chooses, irrespective of very harmful consequences to physical safety or well-being, must be recognized and accepted unless there is clear evidence of the client's incapacity to consent to assistance.

Some elderly persons, however, refuse assistance because they have incorrect information about the nature of the services being offered or the consequences of accepting them. Other elderly persons lack information about ways in which their lives may be made easier or safer through the provision of services. Religious or culturally based convictions about public dependency or accepting charity from strangers may also be reasons for refusing assistance. Experienced clinicians anticipate these kinds of situations and make sure that elderly clients know the professional's role, the services being offered, and what the consequences might be of engaging with the practitioner to receive services.

Some of the common sources of practitioner frustration in working with self-neglecting elderly persons occur because the extent to which an elder understands the harm and dangers of an action or inaction is not clear, there are limited options and resources to provide through intervention, there are many complex and bureaucratic constraints controlling access to resources, informal networks surrounding the client are not providing needed or appropriate assistance, and suspicion prevents an effective practitioner-client relationship from being formed.

Some additional issues often surface during the intervention process. Legal problems and inadequate resources can come into play. Formal care organizations can have admission criteria or eligibility requirements that lengthen the time needed to arrange for services. The informal network that might have once been available may no longer be accessible no matter how great the need of the aged person. Stressed, frightened, and impaired elders often mistrust practitioners whom they consider to be strangers, sometimes for very valid reasons, but they are unable to express this distrust in a direct manner.

The practitioner must assess both the tangible issues of vulnerability, such as obvious physical disability, and the less tangible factors underlying the impaired elder's feelings of self-worth or depression from family rejection. The psychological and social factors in an at-risk elder's life are complex and sometimes subtle. Most potential clients have much inclination and some capacity to exert control over communications when approached by practitioners. It is a challenge, especially when first encountering a very defensive aged person, to maintain maximum flexibility and to adjust the intervention approach to the unique needs and relationship required by the client. The elder, no matter how vulnerable, will greatly influence the process of defining problems and potential needs. Some will want and expect the practitioner to listen directly without questioning them about anything. The majority of what self-neglecting elders reveal to practitioners will come through conversation, not interrogation. Open-ended questions, especially in the beginning stages of the relationship, will consist of general questions that are stated simply and encourage personal reflections and expression of feelings. This information may offer a personalized framework for understanding the client's situation.

MAJOR FACTORS IN ELDER SELF-NEGLECT

It is important to understand what is involved in an elder's effort to cope with lost functional capacity and depleted resources. Our framework defines what is involved in adaptive compensation to manage self-care and discusses the most common individual and environmental factors contributing to self-neglect. Four concepts are helpful to clarify the client's behavior, perception, and motivation as they are related to self-care. *Self-care* refers to actions initiated or tasks performed by the elder as part of the daily routine. *Personal care* is a particular aspect of an elder's daily routine related to physical maintenance. The client's irregular or incomplete or ineffective performance of activities in the daily routine, especially personal care tasks, may reduce *well-being*.

Self-interest is the motivation that keeps an elder trying to perform personal care tasks and complete other more general self-care activities.

Groups and cultures tend to have collective notions of what self-interest behaviors are. When that collective notion is narrow, as is often the case in our culture, individuals whose behaviors do not fit the norms are sometimes inappropriately regarded as lacking in self-interest. Alternatively, in this framework it is assumed that self-interest is a common and normative human motivation; while its expressions may vary, it is the driving force behind an individual's attempts to maintain personal emotional, social, and physical well-being.

THE ADAPTIVE COMPENSATION PROCESS OF SELF-CARE

Most elders act to protect themselves against diverse forms of vulnerability associated with crises and loss. If these cannot be prevented, people find new ways to maintain themselves in the face of altered conditions and circumstances. Many elderly have lost some degree of physical or mental capacity necessary to perform personal care and more general self-care functions. They have made, are making, or need to make some attitudinal shifts and change some behaviors. Modifications in their daily living environments may also be of great importance. Most of the disabled elders who are clients of health-care centers and social service agencies have taken important steps in their own adaptive compensation process as part of their normal aging process. Clinical services can assist elderly clients to take necessary compensating actions that reduce the potential for self-neglect if the clinician understands the complexity of this process.

Table 2.1 illustrates dimensions involved in adaptive compensation for self-care. Elders almost always wish to have control over personal actions and daily life tasks. These are essential to one's sense of personal independence. Each dimension in the chart represents a factor that may be relevant to an elder who is confronted with a major loss of ability and needs to make some adaptive transitions. Almost any major loss has the potential of affecting perceptions because something in the individual or the environment has changed to create one or more deficits in self-care capacity.

Dimension I indicates that an elder questions or reconsiders his or her sense of self when confronted with loss. The person defines that loss as having some impact on personal identity. If the consequences are sufficiently negative, self-esteem is threatened because personal independence is challenged. An effective therapeutic process takes this into account by finding ways that foster rather than reduce client self-esteem.

TABLE 2.1
Dimensions of the Adaptive Compensation Process for Self-Care

I.	Sense of Self — Who am I and what do I need?
II.	Sense of Will — What is my motivation to care for myself and be independent?
III.	Awareness of Capacity — Can I perform tasks and obtain the resources to meet my needs?
IV.	Awareness of Potential — Can I learn a new skill or modify the skill I now retain?
V.	Options in the Environment — Are there resources in my environment that can offer me help?
VI.	Acceptance of Assistance — What actions and activities will I allow others to perform for me?

Dimension II, sense of will, relates to the person's own cognitive and emotional exploration of the loss and ways to manage the impact and consequences. Motivation plays an important role as an aged individual weighs what compensations might be necessary. The more a person's self-esteem is based on independence, the less likely the person is to give up that independence or become dependent on others. Most impaired elderly clients have a day-to-day struggle with self-care but want to maintain control of these functions. A major objective of an intervention effort is to assist the elder who has much pride and determination to keep whatever type and degree of independence is possible in the daily routine, including the resolution of difficulties with self-care tasks.

Dimension III, awareness of capacity, involves the adult's understanding and knowledge of self-care, especially daily personal maintenance tasks. Some clients are clear and accurate about what resources they need to help them complete self-care tasks. Other clients are uncertain or may misjudge what resources are needed to handle tasks. To comprehend realistically what assistance is needed from other people does not mean that assistance is easy to obtain or accept. The service provision process involves helping the client explore self-care needs, and the clinician is challenged to find ways that services can be made available and acceptable.

Dimension IV, awareness of potential, identifies the importance of the elder's learning new skills and/or modifying old behaviors associated with self-care. Cognitive and physical impairments may quickly and drastically disrupt the client's ability to perform self-care functions. This situation may lead to feelings of despair and states of depression that can be eliminated if assistance can be made available with dignity through informal networks and/or community services. Elders gain much satisfaction and a sense of pride when they master new techniques to assist with self-care, such as learning to bathe and dress after suffering paralysis from a stroke. The practitioner needs to be familiar with available community resources. It is important to avoid assuming that clients lack the important potential to learn new skills and to help clients discover this potential.

Dimension V, options in the environment, notes that it is important to consider fully what resources are available in the elder's personal network as well as from formal community resources. Clients who are in crisis or suffering from depression often have difficulty believing that some assistance is available to make daily life better or safer. They may have lost hope. The clinician carries much responsibility to be sensitive to the personal attitudes and feelings, to identify and mobilize the needed supports, and to engage the client in that exploration.

Dimension VI suggests that acceptance of assistance is a vital part of adaptive compensation. If a client perceives that assistance will help to compensate for a loss of functional ability, having the client make use of the resources may not be a major problem. That, however, is often not the case, and a client must be convinced of some potential benefits. Looking for ways to demonstrate the possible value of external assistance is a consistent part of planning and implementing the service plan.

Practitioners may be in a role to assist the elder in transforming a situation of self-neglect into one that is beneficial and leaves the person with a significant amount of self-control. This process can occur through different means. For instance, the practitioner can offer direct information about what resources could be applied to help with self-care without the person giving up all self-control or independence, or the practitioner can facilitate the arrangement of needed resources and, in the process, educate the elder about ways to exercise personal control while taking advantage of the needed services. In almost every situation the practitioner can offer support and ongoing reinforcement for the goal of having as much independence as is realistic. Initially, self-neglecting elders often refuse assistance from other resources because it threatens their sense of self (Dimension I) even though they have very little independence. The clinician needs to understand what the current desire for independence really means to the elder.

Often elders are engaged in adaptive compensation to continue self-care, but their abilities and resources may not be sufficient to prevent conditions of self-neglect because the personal risks being encountered may not be fully understood. The pattern of the onset of individual and environmental risks is important to understand. For example, is the onset of a disability very gradual, and how does this match with the elder's awareness of current capacity (Dimension III).

Clients can be fatalistic about their circumstances sometimes because of the impact on self-perception left by stereotypes about age, disability, and lifestyle patterns (Dimension I). Belief about personal limitations inherent in ageist and ableist stereotypes can exert great influence on the level of motivation to participate in rehabilitation (Dimension II) or to participate in rehabilitation (Dimension IV) or to use available physical environmental supports (Dimension V). In the case of self-neglecting elderly clients, the practitioner should determine if these stereotypes are working to limit a client's view of alternatives or acceptance of resources because of some sense of futility supported by misbelief.

Introducing a therapeutic service and having clients use it is one of the most effective ways to increase understanding of what is or is not a functional limitation (Dimension II) and to gain a realistic sense of self-care capacities that are not easily changed. One approach to deal with a client's strongly held self-perception is to encourage the client to demonstrate to the clinician that tasks can be completed independently. The practitioner must avoid provoking the client's need to defend current self-care abilities.

The clinician is drawn into contact with the elder's informal network if independent performance of self-care tasks is reduced and if that assistance can be made available. Family members and others who are enlisted to help compensate for a client's diminished capacity may need to be informed about the elder's increased need for care and the importance of that assistance being reliable. If family involvement is not in evidence when the clinician first assesses the informal support network, the elder's family members may need to be questioned directly about what assistance they will be willing and able to provide to the client. If the needed assistance is not forthcoming, the client's capacity for adaptive compensation in important areas of self-care is lessened. If at-risk elders attempt to perform tasks beyond their functional ability without the appropriate level of consistent support, the probability of self-neglect increases greatly.

It is very difficult for some elders who are most likely to self-neglect to delegate to others the responsibility for aspects of their life. Not knowing the consequences of that transfer of authority and control may be frightening. Any process of relinquishing control is likely to be one of the most unwelcome aspects of growing old and/or living with disabling conditions, but it is also one of the most important adaptive processes to manage one's vulnerability.

INDIVIDUAL FACTORS CONTRIBUTING TO SELF-NEGLECT

A personal conviction that an elder can be successful at maintaining well-being is central to the motivation for living. Self-neglect may or may not imply loss of interest in self. Loss of interest in self denotes a state in which a person makes little or no attempt to preserve well-being or to manage conditions and events that threaten personal safety. Ironically, it may be the aged person's efforts to maintain a measure of control over personal life circumstances that result in behaviors that are perceived and defined by clinicians as self-neglect. Although the bases for self-worth, which most elders derive from their social roles and relationships, as well as their contributions to the outer world, may narrow with the aging process or diminish from disability, most at-risk elders do continue to maintain some major interest in their personal well-being.

The most pervasive way this interest gets expressed is through motivation to sustain independent self-care as long as possible. Most elders want to believe they can control functions and perform tasks necessary for survival. Self-care activities are very important expressions of self-interest. Self-care activities may be the last area of functioning over which personal control can be exerted, so as a result clients want and need to believe themselves capable of the maximum amount of independent self-maintenance. When questioned, elders often find it difficult to admit limitations. The inability to perform self-care tasks, combined with lack of recognition of or admission to these limitations, is the most common personal reason for elder self-neglect.

Without recognizing or admitting limitations, at-risk elders can eventually suffer serious, if not fatal, consequences from self-neglect, especially when their environment does not offer the needed resources or when they cannot accept available needed resources. Professional intervention might be unnecessary if all aged people were capable of self-care tasks sufficient to assure their well-being and if, when assistance was needed, they could receive help without fear, loss of dignity, and loss of personal control. Unfortunately, these are not the real conditions that face many elderly persons.

Each individual has a personal sense of well-being that is not always based on prevailing views about the way self-care tasks should be performed. Many older people with major and multiple impairments continue to perceive that their self-interest is best protected if they control self-care decisions and activities. If that perception is held by the elder, it influences the definition of personal needs and self-care capacities and may affect willingness to accept assistance. However, a person's belief that he or she is acting out of self-interest to perform activities beyond actual capacity sets the stage for potential self-neglect. Clinicians often differ with clients over self-control issues; there are different perceptions about the client's capacity to complete self-care tasks and about adequate management of basic needs.

ENVIRONMENTAL FACTORS CONTRIBUTING TO SELF-NEGLECT

Conditions of self-neglect may be increased or decreased and sometimes created by environmental factors that surround and directly impact the elder, so in many cases environmental conditions become a focus of the assessment and later intervention. The impact of environmental factors can often be greater than individual conditions influencing the self-neglect. Among the environmental factors most likely to affect individual conditions are those within informal networks and the immediate social environment such as family members, friends, and neighbors. The formal network of organized service, either available or unavailable to the elder at risk, are environmental factors that become directly related to situations of self-neglect. The inaccessibility of formal supports needed by elders is one of the most influential conditions increasing the potential of self-neglect.

Among the services most needed, but sometimes not available, are medical care, transportation, financial assistance, nutrition, in-home services, respite care, specialized housing, metal health counseling, adult day care programs, inpatient rehabilitation programs, affordable nursing homes, and socialization programs for those with disabilities. Even when these resources and services exist in a community, they may be inaccessible for financial reasons including eligibility requirements for third-party reimbursement. Environmental factors can make a dramatic difference in the degree of risk of self-neglect.

TREATING SELF-NEGLECT CASES

Many cases of self-neglect represent sources of exasperation for the practitioner, and the client frequently evaluates those in a position to be of greatest help as though they were a threatening adversary. Practitioners offering service options to clients must understand the meanings of these options for the client and be sensitive to ways that service utilization, once the notion of accepting assistance is agreed upon, may reduce the actual or perceived degree of client control over life circumstances. Sometimes the practitioner will devote considerable effort to mediate the control that formal service assistance exerts on the client. Clinical experience suggests that no standard approach can guarantee that a practitioner-client relationship can be easily formulated with elders at greatest risk of self-neglect. However, some general guidelines are useful to follow.

Forming the Relationship

Often the relationship between practitioner and client will require that each party take on roles and functions of different levels of independence and authority. The greater the amount of distress and danger experienced by the client, the more likely it is the practitioner experiences a sense of urgency to provide immediate intervention. Although this sense of responsibility may be appropriate, to move too quickly can reduce the likelihood of framing an effective relationship because the client may be too confused or frightened to accept the offer of an interdependent, not dependent, relationship with the practitioner. Practitioners, especially those who are expected to have the quick and permanent solution for elders in crisis, may sometimes have to weigh community pressure for immediate intervention against the slower relationship-building process with the client.

The importance of the elder maintaining the power of decision making may force the practitioner to spend considerable time in collaborative exploration and the selection of alternatives with the specific intention of increasing client trust and maintenance of client choice about options. With self-neglecting elders, the perception of control and the self-esteem related to it are essential conditions for well-being.

The Assessment Process

Assuming that the major goal of assessment is to determine the individual's risk of self-neglect, including environmental correlates, core areas of assessment include impairment levels, economic resource adequacy, safety in the residential space, availability of formal and informal resource networks, adequacy of the assistance provided by networks, the extent of physical and social isolation, depression, cognitive orientation, and related biopsychological problems. Whenever possible assessment should include input from other formal service contacts and informal network associations that are thought to be relevant to risk determination. The focus of the assessment is primarily the present situation; however, this emphasis should not preclude attention to either past or future as it relates to client vulnerability. Many self-neglecting elders have been engaged in a long and weary process of adapting to decreased capacities, lessened financial security, and a reduced social network. They may have forfeited any hope of personal security and may also be experiencing progressive physical and cognitive losses that affect their perceptions of personal capacities and opportunities.

Planning the Foundation for Ongoing Services

Forming a relationship that progresses slowly and allows the worker and a self-neglecting elder to form trusting and caring bonds is one of the most effective components of individual counseling or case work. But many barriers may make this impossible if the elderly client is first seen in a crisis situation. Based on observations of social workers in the process of providing services to clients, we have noted several patterns. First, crisis intervention will be useful in resolving emergency problems that arise in the client's life. Perhaps the crisis will be directly associated with the self-neglect, but crisis problem solving does little to redirect the elder's patterns toward more effective self-reliance. Our second observation is that the relationship, if established on a solid foundation of trust, does become the vehicle for personal change from more to less self-neglecting behavior. This may occur because the elder feels he or she has finally built a relationship with someone who will listen to wishes and plans without passing quick judgment on inadequacy or limitations. A mutual process of considering options that the client perceives as desirable can also extend into the client's being more willing to accept suggestions made by the practitioner.

Being an Advocate for the Client

Clients often have no frame of reference to understand the practitioner's desire to be a helpful advocate. Certainly some elderly clients have been promised assistance from a formal agency that has not resulted in the anticipated services the client was hoping to attain. Most of them, however, have little experience with a stranger offering to confront large bureaucratic systems that are not client friendly. They may not know how to interpret a practitioner's willingness to confront the Medicaid eligibility process or the Title VIII public housing manager on the client's behalf. A lifetime of relying only on personal resources or never knowing about a relationship that does not demand payment for every favor has not prepared clients for this unfamiliar relationship. It is easy to overlook the consequences of a lifetime of socialization that requires self-reliance rather than cooperation and shared responsibilities.

Conclusion

This framework has been presented at a general level in order to provide the greatest applicability of its components across different professional practice areas. It is not intended to be a prescription for in-depth psychotherapeutic counseling or personal health care. Rather it was prepared as a means to share the results gathered from extensive field work on social service delivery to self-neglecting and other-neglected older persons.

The economic, medical, and social services implications of self-neglecting behavior among elders are often obvious, and practical solutions to individual problems are frequently readily apparent. However, the effective management of certain difficult cases, the development of fair-minded and compassionate policies, and insight into self-neglect as a societal issue all require a broader, more critical, and more structured view.

II

SYSTEMS CONSIDERATIONS

3

Ethical Issues in Working with Self-Neglect

Stephen J. Cutler and William A. Tisdale

In this chapter, we describe a tentative framework for ethical analysis of some issues surrounding self-neglecting elders. First of all, we suggest several moral principles and derivative rules that seem relevant to the recognition and resolution of geriatric self-neglect. Then, we present and discuss four case summaries, each illustrating one or more ethical concerns encountered in everyday practice. Finally, we propose some decision-making strategies and criteria that professionals (and others) might employ in dealing with instances of self-neglect among the aged.

MAJOR ETHICAL PRINCIPLES PERTAINING TO SELF-NEGLECT: AUTONOMY, BENEFICENCE, AND JUSTICE

In cases of self-neglecting elders (and in instances of elder abuse and frailty more generally), we often face a dilemma, which Quinn (1985, p. 23) characterizes as one of freedom versus safety, one which, she notes, "bedevils practitioners who work with the frail elderly. They are trained to intervene and help solve their clients' problems, and by temperament they wish to be of service. It also concerns those who give priority to the rights of all adults to be free [of] governmental interference."

When threats to an individual's well-being, internally or externally produced, are present, our professional training and humanitarian impulses quite naturally lead us to wish to intervene so as to restore persons to optimum levels of physical, social, or economic functioning. "Caregivers," Dubler (1987, p. 140) writes, "are trained to decide and to intervene, not to negotiate, mediate, and withhold." In cases of willful self-neglect, however, a desire to remove barriers to well-being may run directly counter to the individual's wishes. At the most fundamental level, then, this clash in values between freedom and safety reflects the tension between two basic ethical principles: autonomy and beneficence. These two principles almost invariably come into play and often into conflict in instances of self-neglect.

Autonomy

The principle of autonomy, rooted in the deontological tradition of Kant, emphasizes respect for persons and holds that each individual can establish and realize his or her life plan without interference so long as the rights of others are not denied. According to Collopy (1988, p. 10), autonomy is understood as a cluster of notions including self-determination, freedom, independence, liberty of choice, and action. In its most general terms, autonomy signifies control of decision making and other activity by the individual. It refers to human agency free of outside intervention and interference. Or, as Wetle (1985, p. 30) puts it, "Individual autonomy refers to the individual's right to make decisions that are voluntary and intentional, and not the result of coercion, duress or undue influence." Subject to qualifications that we note later, autonomy stresses a person's right to self-determination, the right to choose freely from among the available options, and the right to carry out that choice (Dworkin, 1976; Gadow, 1980).

Thus, autonomy accords the highest priority to freedom. If individuals are capable of making decisions, if they are aware of and understand the consequences of those decisions, and if the welfare of others is not at issue, respect for persons as autonomous agents would lead us to adopt a hands-off stance toward self-neglecting elders. Our position would be one of noninterference in the course of action they have chosen, even if that course of action, in our judgment, is detrimental to their physical, social, or economic well-being.

When we move beyond a general statement of the principle of autonomy to its application in cases of self-neglecting elders, important issues and questions emerge. Here we consider two of them. Respecting a person's autonomy presumes that the individual is competent to make decisions and that the decisions are voluntary and informed (Kapp and Bigot, 1985, pp. 23–32).

Competency, an individual's mental or intellectual capacity to perform certain functions or particular acts, is an especially critical issue in dealing with the problem of self-neglect in elders. Questions of intellectual capability arise in all age groups, especially in medical and legal contexts, but they are especially common among isolated, ill, or institutionalized elderly (Stanley, Stanley, Guido, and Garvin, 1988). Chronic diseases and disabilities, such as dementia, stroke, and heart failure, may compromise higher mental functions. Many treatments, such as those prescribed for depression and high blood pressure, blunt intellectual performance in some patients. Social isolation, marginal economic status, and prolonged institutionalization can all affect judgment and insight. Equally important, health professionals, families, and others may erroneously assume that advanced age itself dulls the intellect.

The definition of competency remains basically legal, for determination of competency is a judicial decision based on testimony and assessment of health professionals and others. The President's Commission for the Study of Ethical Problems in Medicine and Biomedical and Behavioral Research (1982) determined, in concept, that competency involved possession of a set of values and goals, the ability to communicate and understand information, and the ability to reason and deliberate about one's choices. At a more practical level, most working definitions of competency parallel that of *Grannum* (1967), where the court stated that "the test [is] whether the person in question ... possessed sufficient mind or reason to enable him to understand the nature, the terms and the effects of the transaction." In essence, the self-neglecting older person could be declared legally incompetent if those concerned for his or her welfare showed that he or she could not grasp the nature of the threat and its possible impact on his or her welfare.

A rather special concern for issues of competency often relates to critical decisions about health care. Here, instead of concerns about capacity to manage property or assets, the dilemma involves decisions about appropriate therapy for symptoms, diseases, and disabilities that threaten the autonomous agent. The search continues for some universal criteria of competency, but the wide diversity of medical conditions and related decisions makes success quite unlikely.

Competency, then, is an elusive notion, both conceptually and operationally (Culver, 1985; High, 1987; Meisel, Roth, and Lidz, 1977). Legal and clinical definitions may differ; assessment can be imprecise; and competency varies across functional domains and fluctuates over time. One must be careful not to view competency as a categorical, either-or construct.

Most health-related competency questions arise when personal consent is required for a clinical procedure, typically when a geriatric patient refuses a test or treatment recommended by a physician. (Decisions to accept medical advice — even unsound advice — are rarely questioned.) Recent medical, legal, and ethical writings have clarified, but not resolved, many of the issues involved in informed consent. In general, assurance of valid and informed consent to medical treatment involves the three variables of full and adequate information, legal competency, and demonstrated understanding of the issues involved; one precondition — truly voluntary decision making; and one consequence — a firm decision (Meisel, Roth, and Lidz, 1977).

Beneficence

Standing in potentially sharp contrast to the principle of autonomy is the principle of beneficence. Derived from the utilitarian theories of Bentham and Mill, beneficence stresses a rather different set of obligations. According to Beauchamp and Childress (1989, p. 195), beneficence "requires the *provision* of benefits (including the prevention and removal of harm as well as the promotion of welfare) . . . and a *balancing* of benefits and harms." As such, it sets the stage and provides the moral underpinnings for paternalism — the "refusal to accept or acquiesce in another person's wishes, choices, and actions for that person's own benefit" (Childress, 1982, p. 13), especially when it is deemed that the harm(s) resulting from an individual's decisions and actions will outweigh the good(s).

Whereas autonomy is primarily concerned with the freedom of the individual to make decisions, beneficence emphasizes a person's welfare and safety. Autonomy concerns itself with individual liberty; beneficence stresses the realization of benefits for the individual. The former argues that certain principles, for example the right to self-determination, should not be overridden or compromised, even if harmful consequences for the self-neglecting person are certain. The latter suggests that interests must be balanced, that harms and benefits must be weighed, and that the proper course of action, which is in the best interests of the individual, might not always be what that person would have wished for himself or herself. With autonomy, the principal locus of decision making is with the affected individual. With beneficence, other actors (for example, profes-sionals and family members) lay claim to decision-making rights.

Beneficence requires that one help others by promoting their welfare and preventing injury or harm. Most public social, economic, and health-care programs take their moral foundation from this imperative. Implicit in the concept of beneficence is a utilitarian calculus involving a balance of good (health, happiness, or fulfillment) and harm (illness, suffering, or neglect). Will a particular intervention produce, on balance, more good than harm?

Many societal interventions or actions taken on behalf of self-neglecting older persons are obviously correct and morally justified: the targets of real estate swindlers should be prevented from squandering their life savings; a demented widow must not be allowed to live in an unheated hovel; and the near-blind retiree should not drive on crowded interstate highways. Other equally well-motivated interventions, as we shall see in the cases that follow, are less purely beneficent and raise a basic — and bothersome — question: Whose welfare (benefit)? Whose injury (cost)?

Physicians and other health-care professionals, lawyers, social workers, and others in the personal service sector traditionally have a duty to individual patients/clients. As their advocates, these professionals make decisions that (they hope) benefit particular elders. When cost-benefit assessments suggest individual gain or benefit at some cost to society, most professionals choose the personal good. Public servants, such as Medicaid administrators, city health workers, and housing authority workers may, predictably, assign very different weights to individual cost-benefit values.

Answers to cost-benefit equations are usually simple when the older person understands the relative benefits and potential costs involved. Again, however, serious ethical and legal problems arise when dementia, depression, or other disabilities compromise the person's judgment and powers of comprehension. All too often, a well-meaning (beneficent) advocate intercedes with opinions, decisions, or actions presumed to be in the recipient's best interest even though the person in question has other wishes. Decisions made or actions taken on behalf of a recipient against his or her wishes constitute paternalism, reflecting a sort of "father knows best" presumption of wisdom.

Ethicists have written extensively about the tensions between autonomy and paternalism. Some, like John Stuart Mill, insist that autonomy or individual liberty must be respected in all instances except when a particular action would cause real harm to others. Other writers accept a more invasive or directive form of paternalistic intervention, arguing that the affairs of a compromised or incompetent individual may properly be managed by a beneficent person or agency (so-called weak paternalism). Few philosophers favor strong paternalism, that is the overriding of a competent and informed person's wishes about his or her affairs. But older persons, especially those who are eccentric, infirm, isolated, or poor, are frequently subjected to misguided paternalistic manipulations (Cohen, 1988): the careless widow has her bank account taken over by her oversolicitous daughter; an anxious son persuades a physician to recommend cancellation of his father's driver's license; a vigorous, retired 80-year-old woman is told by her children that it is unsafe for her to live alone in her lake cottage.

These and many other interventions, however well-intentioned and basically beneficent in nature, do threaten the independence and dignity of the older person. Would-be benefactors, whether individuals or agencies, should analyze each action and decision proposed for the welfare of a client, determine the client's wishes, values, and priorities, and weigh carefully the possible impact of each effort on the recipient. As far as possible, paternalistic actions, as we emphasize later, must be limited in both degree of imposition and duration.

Justice

Yet a third ethical framework pertains to the situation of self-neglecting elders. This is the principle of justice, which directs attention to the just, proper, or fair allocation of scarce resources. Considerations of justice generally occur at two levels. The first concerns itself with justice at the macrolevel: how should a society's scarce resources be distributed when there are competing claims on those resources? What is the proper allocation of the federal budget for defense, for health, for social services? And within these areas, how should limited resources be distributed? When the fiscal pie is not large enough to provide for all worthy programs, how should the claims of programs and services for needy children be weighed against the claims of programs and services for needy elders?

Issues related to justice, however, are not restricted to questions about the macroallocation of resources. Also of relevance is the issue of microallocation. After decisions have been made about the proper distribution of resources among competing programs and services, it still remains to decide which individuals or groups of individuals are eligible to be recipients of those resources. The United States has chosen to make treatment of end-stage renal dialysis available to persons regardless of their age. In contrast, Great Britian has elected to exclude older persons from treatment in end-stage renal dialysis programs (Moskop, 1987; Office of Technology Assessment, 1987).

The issue of justice has some relevance to the situation of self-neglecting elders. Childress (1982, p. 15) notes that the consequences of a "person's actions might impose unfair burdens on others by requiring extensive resources to which members of the community have contributed." Is it legitimate to weigh such a consideration when balancing the duties implied by beneficence against an individual's right to exercise autonomous decision making? In times of fiscal constraints and limited service resources, is it proper to take into account cost-savings that may be realized from paternalistic interventions in the lives of self-neglecting elders, even if those interventions may come at the expense of compromising personal autonomy?

Although few of us would question the Aristotelian concept of pure justice — equals ought to be treated equally — we often question its particular applications. The derivative or secondary principle of distributive justice, or the justified and proper distribution of benefits among individuals in society, is most relevant to the problems posed by self-neglecting elders. This principle suggests that like cases be treated alike and different cases be treated differently in direct proportion to the differences between them. As noted by Hume (1983), however, ethical difficulties arise with just and equal treatment when the goods or services being sought and distributed are in short supply. Conflicts and difficulties emerge in designing and administering just or fair distribution schemes for the dependent elderly, for no two cases seem exactly alike (or equal) in terms of age, type and level of need, probable benefits, and associated costs. Because totally just decisions of this sort can rarely be reached, perhaps the main goal of providers should be to avoid arbitrary inequality in selecting recipients of economic, social, or medical benefits. In assigning subsidized apartments to low-income elders, for example, educational level should not be considered a crucial variable; when hospital beds are in short supply, personal cleanliness should not be a criterion for admission; and the demented, self-neglecting widower should not be penalized by clinic physicians for his poor medical compliance.

A final dimension of applied justice relates to willfully self-neglectful persons: is an older (or younger) person morally obliged to protect and promote his or her own health? Should society provide the same benefits to a knowingly self-neglectful elder that are offered to others who work toward their own health and welfare? Despite the arguments of Sider and Clements (1984), most ethicists do not consider obligation to self or to health promotion a moral principle. Although the self-neglectful but competent older person may tax the tolerance and resources of medical, social, and other types of agencies, denial of appropriate benefits and services rarely leads to reform and may, in fact, invite disaster.

CASE STUDIES

Case #1: Self-Neglect in the Caregiver

Mrs. A, a 75-year-old retired teacher, lives in her small home with her husband, a 78-year-old retired lawyer, who has moderately advanced Alzheimer's disease. She consulted a geriatrician for advice about his increasingly disruptive and demanding behavior. Once a successful, hard-driving government investigator, her husband has well-documented primary dementia, presumably SDAT. Over the last three years, he has become progressively forgetful, disoriented, and depressed, with recent increasing agitation, sleeplessness, and wandering. At present, despite brief trials of sedatives and neouleptic therapy, his behavior has become almost uncontrolled: his wife dresses him each morning, with maximum coaxing, only to have him disrobe and refuse to cooperate until she chooses a new set of clothes. He frequently refuses meals, then consumes large quantities of food in a few minutes. Although he accompanies her on shopping trips, he often wanders off in stores and parking lots; twice the police were called to search for him. Many nights are sleepless for the couple, as Mr. A paces about the living room and turns lights on and off.

Mrs. A, in relating these dramatic events and describing her failed attempts to control his behavior, made no reference to her own plight — "George has always needed my help, and I've never had to ask for outside help or advice." It emerged that she had refused any offers of assistance and respite from family, friends, and neighbors — "We manage . . . I am the only one who understands his problem." She had not had a day alone for more than two years; she no longer attended church, feeling the services upset her husband; she fired one homemaker after a single visit — "George became frantic, and I can manage now that we have locked up the garage and the cellar." She rarely got more than two consecutive hours of sleep at night — "Of course I am tired, but we can nap anytime during the next day." She made passing reference to her own health — "My blood pressure and thyroid trouble have not caused any difficulties in more than a year."

After two hours of discussion, she thanked the consultant, eventually refusing all suggestions of day care or other assistance — "If that is all you have to offer, we will just make it on our own."

Commentary

Three points deserve emphasis. First, self-neglect or health-related problems were not mentioned when Mrs. A was referred to the geriatrician by a family friend. In fact, she was praised for her devotion and unselfish care. Thus, self-neglect may not be apparent to all observers. Older persons often willingly and knowingly sacrifice personal care, comfort, and independence in their efforts to provide for a family member or close friend. The boundaries between selfless generosity and harmful self-denial are often vague and indistinct. The behaviors and practices constituting self-neglect may be open to disagreement.

Second, the situation of Mrs. A demonstrates that the harmful effects of neglectful behavior often have profound implications for others as well as for the self-neglecting individual. Mrs. A was finally persuaded that further neglect of her hypertension could result in a crippling stroke or heart attack, events that would necessitate placing her husband in a nursing home. As shown later in this chapter, the decision to intervene directly may hinge on the likelihood that others are affected by the elder's self-neglecting behaviors.

Finally, this case shows that it is often difficult to design and provide effective and humane intervention, especially when the neglectful person is basically competent and both well-motivated and well-meaning. Mrs. A saw "outside help" as a denial of her own loving care and competence, and she refused day care as both too expensive and too demeaning for her husband.

Case #2: The Community Costs of Self-Neglect

Mr. B, an 80-year-old retired laborer, basically healthy except for moderately severe chronic lung disease, has a unique, slowly progressive, and untreatable form of amnesia, presumably the result of chronic alcohol abuse. He is alert, oriented, generally rational; he is articulate and socially at ease; he has excellent remote memory, but has essentially no recent memory or recall — he cannot remember names, numbers, instructions, or events beyond 10 or 15 minutes.

At present, he lives alone in a one-room studio apartment in subsidized housing for the elderly, eats his noon meal at a nearby senior center, just barely managing to keep enough food on hand for evening snacks. With maximum assistance from his daughters, who live five and ten miles distant, his apartment is cleaned, his clothes are washed, and his few bills are paid regularly.

However, his medical care has been chaotic and disastrous. He requires two long-acting capsules of Theophylline each day, and no safe system of delivery has been devised despite efforts of several physicians, the Home Health agency, the Office on Aging, the Mental Health Service, and several local hospital workers. Given seven days' medication supply, he takes all 14 capsules in 24 hours or less ("Did I take the morning dose?"), and he has been hospitalized twice in the past year with acute intoxication. Given two to six capsules, he takes all at once, then develops wheezing, cough, and a panic reaction a day or so later ("No one left the pills"). He had visited the emergency room on more than 20 occasions in the last two months. Neither the local housing director nor the senior center worker can assume medical responsibilities; the family is exhausted by endless trips and around-the-clock telephone calls; mental health workers visit the apartment, only to find that Mr. B is wandering about town. After several formal evaluations, his physician persuaded the probate judge that Mr. B was "medically incompetent," but his daughters do not have authority to force a change in residence.

At a recent long-term care conference, Mr. B repeated his insistence that he live independently, pointing out that he had never been arrested, accepted full responsibility for his own safety, and threatened to "disown" his daughters if they forced him to move.

Commentary

Several issues are raised by this case and by Mr. B's grossly self-neglectful practices. As we will note later in this chapter, even the marginally competent person may insist on — and retain — a high degree of autonomy so long as no harm comes to others. Although severely handicapped by his defective memory, Mr. B demanded and received independence in housing and other social functions. The probate judge carefully delineated his area of incompetence, pointing out that the risks otherwise involved in independent living were acceptable by usual standards.

The case of Mr. B also shows that the line between beneficent support and paternalistic intervention may be a fine one, open to dispute and disagreement. Convinced that he was a danger to himself, a few workers favored legal action to force him into a more structured and protective environment. A majority, however, sided with the judge, feeling that direct manipulation of Mr. B and his lifestyle should be limited to factors that posed an immediate threat to his health and safety.

In addition, this case highlights an economic or resource-allocation issue. A conservative estimate placed the monthly costs of Mr. B's use and misuse of medical and support services at about $2,500. Increasingly, caregivers and agencies are questioning the ethical and economic implications of self-neglecting behaviors that consume vital community resources.

Case #3: Personal Preferences versus Professional Judgment

Miss C is 78 years old, single, and has run an 800-acre ranch for the last 50 years. She has at times hired part-time laborers, but essentially she has taken care of all operations herself. Although she is no longer able to ride horseback, she gets around in a four-wheel-drive jeep. During the last five years, she has had circulatory problems in her right leg due in part to an injury she received from being thrown from a horse six years before. On a visit to her local physician it becomes clear that the circulation is seriously compromised and that an amputation will be necessary. Miss C refuses. She looks at the situation this way: She has lived her entire life on her own, and she figures she can take care of her leg by herself. Anyway, if things go badly from the infection, she has lived a full life.

Her physician always considered Miss C somewhat peculiar and has come to worry about her judgment over the last seven years, during which period she has become even more idiosyncratic, uncooperative, and hostile toward those who attempt to help her. The physician visited her house once and found it for the most part full of old boxes, newspapers, and two dozen cats. The physician believes that for her own good Miss C should be declared incompetent and forced to have her right leg amputated. He points out that she can very likely learn to use a prosthesis to get around her house and even to drive her jeep. (This case is drawn from Brody and Englehardt, 1987, p. 337.)

Commentary

Miss C's physician was properly concerned about a key issue in the care of many self-neglecting persons: that is, her competence to make critical decisions. On the one hand, Miss C's eccentric behavior and seemingly unwise judgments about health care did not, of themselves, constitute incompetency in a legal sense. On the other hand, failure to recognize and document true incompetency, or inability to understand particular decisions and their consequences, could lead to further neglect, disability, and even death. The basic question is, "Who decides who decides?"

Case #4: Preserving the Right of Self-Determination

Mrs. D, a 75-year-old woman with chronic obstructive lung disease and advanced peripheral arterial insufficiency, was transferred to a nursing home for terminal care. It soon became apparent that her right foot was gangrenous, but the patient, who had undergone arteriogram studies in the hospital, refused surgical care or amputation — "I just dread it ... I would be deformed and crippled." After extensive consultation, several family discussions, and one legal consultation, the staff agreed that the patient was competent to direct her own care and that her decision should be respected. Terminal care plans were written, with emphasis on support and comfort.

About two weeks later, the patient began to refuse solid food — "Nothing tastes good ... I am too tired to eat" — and within a week she refused most offers of fluids — "No appeal ... why fight to prolong the misery?" Her daughter, who had cared for Mrs. D at home for years, became anxious and angry with the staff: "She can refuse major surgery, but she cannot just commit suicide. She has become irrational and confused, so how can she make this terrible decision? You can't let her suffer and die from lack of water — that is inhuman and immoral."

The staff was evenly divided over the proper course of action. Many nurses felt the patient was quite lucid and competent, pointing out that her refusal of fluids was consistent with her prior refusal of surgery. Others were convinced that she had become irrational and depressed, arguing that simple dietary support was not invasive and that vigorous enteral or parenteral fluid and nutrient replacement could, in a matter of a week, restore her comfort and desire to live.

After several exhausting conferences, the daughter and nursing home staff agreed to the following plan: Mrs. D would dictate a list of foods and fluids she might accept; small portions would be offered every hour while she was awake; a pain medication and a mild tranquilizer would be given regularly; no further laboratory or fluid balance study would be ordered.

Still taking only sips of fluids, the patient lapsed into a coma a week later, and she died quietly three days later.

Commentary

In the case of Mrs. D, two important issues were raised by the reactions of the daughter and the nursing staff during her terminal illness. First, Mrs. D's would-be benefactors, all deeply concerned and committed to do the right thing for her, disagreed on several basic facts. Some believed her to be competent and rational; others considered her depressed, confused, and incapable of making proper decisions about her treatment. Time and again, individuals and agencies charged with promoting the medical, economic, or social welfare of elderly clients disagree on the very nature and dimensions of self-neglect and, predictably, on the appropriate intervention.

Second, the intervention or corrective action sought by the daughter, the simple provision of food and water, seemed minimal and noninvasive. Nonetheless, this step would have denied Mrs. D's autonomy and overridden what seemed to be her expressed wishes about her dying. Many people concerned about self-neglecting elders justify their uninvited interventions with talk of "minimal," "temporary," and "until she is stronger" (Collopy, 1988). Perceptive older people often note and remember this first unwelcomed incursion that started their slide toward total dependence.

ETHICAL CONSIDERATIONS AND INTERVENTION STRATEGIES

This section applies in a more formal manner the ethical principles and issues previously discussed to the situation of self-neglecting elders. We will attempt to develop some tentative decision-making strategies, which may be of assistance to practitioners confronted with older persons who exhibit self-neglecting behaviors. We hasten to add, however, that these guidelines are perhaps most applicable to clear-cut cases. As in all such matters, the proper course of action is clearest at the extremes. Yet self-neglect, as was emphasized in Chapters 1 and 2, is complex and only rarely reducible to straightforward answers upon which all involved parties agree.

Any consideration of possible intervention in the case of a self-neglecting elder must begin with a judgment about the person's competence. Setting aside for the moment the issue of whether others are likely to be affected by the self-neglecting individual's behaviors, when an older person is knowingly self-neglectful, but clearly competent to exercise decision making, the principle of autonomy should prevail.

In the part that concerns only himself, his independence is, of right, absolute. Over himself, over his own body and mind, the individual is sovereign (Mill, 1863, p. 23). A competent individual's failure to exercise self-care when the welfare of others is not at issue, however regrettable this may be to outside observers, is not sufficient to justify paternalistic intervention (Chadwick and Russell, 1989; Dubler, 1988). Persons who possess all relevant information about the possible or likely outcomes of their actions, who are able to deliberate rationally about alternatives, and who have reached a voluntary and informed decision about the course of action (or inaction) they wish to pursue based on their values and preferences should have that decision respected. As Arras (1987, p. 65) notes, "the possibility of self-inflicted risks of harm cannot suffice, by itself, to undercut a person's presumed capacity to make decisions." This is true regardless of the severity of harm that may befall the individual.

Perhaps the clearest illustration of this situation is the case of Miss C discussed above. Without treatment, the circulatory problems in her leg will most likely lead to her death. Yet, aside from some seeming eccentricities, nothing in the case seems to indicate decisional incapacity. She has been a fiercely independent woman throughout her life and has successfully managed a large ranch. No other persons would appear to be affected by the course of action she has chosen.

To say, however, that autonomy must be respected in this and in similar cases is not to suggest that practitioners and caregivers should abandon all concern for the self-neglecting elder's welfare. Jackson and Youngner (1979) present several examples from clinical situations where a patient's initial preference to have treatment withheld or discontinued was ultimately reversed by the patient himself. Continuing to monitor the individual's well-being, providing relevant information, and being alert to any signs of a change in wishes do not represent unnecessary intrusion.

The situation is more complicated when the actions of the self-neglectful elder have consequences for others. Of course, one can conceive of circumstances in which all of those directly involved are competent, do not wish to infringe on the elder's right to self-determination, and are willing to endure any harms that may befall them. By extension, then, the principle of autonomy would again dictate that the self-neglectful elder's wishes be honored in such circumstances. However, when the others who are implicated are unaware of the consequences, unwilling to suffer them, or when the other person's competence is somehow compromised, there is reason to intervene. In such instances, we confront the difficult problem where "the severity and likelihood of potential hazards to others must be weighed against the importance of respecting the . . . [self-neglecting elder's] . . . preference or spoken choice" (Zuckerman, 1987, p. 68).

Among the cases presented earlier in this chapter, that of Mrs. A is instructive in this regard. By refusing all offers of assistance, she made her seriously demented husband largely dependent on her ability to care for him. She has taken upon herself the responsibility of protecting him from harm and securing his safety and well-being. Yet, Mrs. A is neglecting her own health. If this neglect of her own physical welfare leads to impairment, her husband would then be placed at some considerable risk. Even though no one has seriously questioned her competence, her actions could ultimately bring harm to Mr. A. Thus, some form of limited paternalistic intervention seems warranted in this instance.

We recognize, of course, that this is a situation in which the potential harm to Mr. A is clear and potentially a direct result of Mrs. A's self-neglect. An identifiable individual may be placed at risk. A comparable situation would be the case of a competent elder whose self-neglectful practices with gas or electric appliances place neighbors in an apartment building in potential jeopardy. In other instances, however, the harms may be real, but less consequential, or the affected others may not be as readily identifiable. The older person living in willful and self-imposed squalor may cause considerable consternation among neighbors, but whether real or perceived threats to property values can justify intervention remains a question. Putting aside the issue of Mr. B's competence, in the second case described earlier, the effects on others seem largely to be indirect and of an economic nature. Again, it is questionable whether excessive health care expenditures for Mr. B alone justify intervention.

In the situations just described, we have made the simplifying assumption that the self-neglecting elder is competent and evidences decisional capacity. So long as others are uninvolved, or so long as they are competent and willing to put themselves at risk as a consequence of the self-neglecting elder's behavior, we have little basis for infringements on the right to self-determination. Just as clear is the morally permissible, even the morally required, course of action when the elder's self-neglect is the product of incompetence or decisional incapacity. When older persons are grossly or obviously incompetent, relatively few ethical or legal problems interfere with preventing and correcting self-neglecting behavior. Regardless of the magnitude of the actual or potential harm, and regardless of whether others are affected, an older person whose competence is clearly diminished has a right to the protection and security that can be provided by beneficent, paternalistic intervention.

Yet, as we have noted earlier, competence is not an "all or nothing," an "either-or," concept (Culver, 1985). Beyond the extreme cases of uncontested competence or uncontested incompetence lie numerous situations where the decisional capacity of individuals is variable or questionable. A person may be competent in some domains but not in others. Competence may be intermittent and fluctuate over time. Thus, the most difficult cases of self-neglect involve older persons with inconstant evidence of impaired or diminished competence or "borderline" individuals who suffer from emotional illness, who have sustained brain damage (for example, Alzheimer's disease or stroke), or who manifest bizarre or eccentric behavior. In these instances, a two-step general strategy should be employed to ensure respect and fairness. Would-be benefactors should try to shed light on potentially reversible causes of reduced competence: failing or changing mental status should be assessed; medical conditions that affect thinking and behavior should be investigated; and obvious social or economic stresses that could affect perception and behavior should be noted and, if possible, corrected before outside standards are imposed on the self-neglecting person. Treatment of crippling depression often transforms the elderly patient; provision of transportation may liberate an elderly recluse; and visits by Senior Companions have energized many older shut-ins.

All too often, however, self-neglecting old persons prove to have significant, often progressive cognitive losses caused by Alzheimer's dementia, brain damage from stroke, and the like. Even in these instances, denial of autonomy and assumption of control cannot be based on limited observations, personal judgment, and presumptions of authority. Family members should be sought for both direct assistance and their possible insights into the older person's previous values and goals. Any clinical condition should be evaluated and treated by competent medical professionals. Only after such steps have been taken should concerned family and professionals consider petitioning the court for a decision about competency in health and other affairs and for a decision about appropriate interventions.

However, the mode or form of intervention also needs to be addressed. Beneficence, when morally justified or required, may take many forms. To the extent possible, paternalistic interventions should be chosen so as to minimize intrusions and retain maximum autonomy, given the circumstances of a particular self-neglecting elder.

In general, interventions can be arrayed along a continuum ranging from the most intrusive and restrictive (representing the suspension of civil rights and liberties) to the least intrusive and restrictive (representing minimal or limited threats to autonomy). Kapp and Bigot (1985) note several of these mechanisms. Involuntary commitment or hospitalization can be used to institutionalize persons who, by virtue of mental illness, represent a threat either to others or to themselves. Less restrictive in terms of institutionalization, but equally consequential for civil liberties, is the use of guardianships (Schmidt, 1985) and conservatorships. Both require a judicial determination of incompetence and both involve the appointment of someone to make decisions on behalf of the incapacitated elder. The difference, however, is that "conservatorship usually means the appointment of someone with power over the property of another, and guardianship means the appointment of someone with power over the property and person of another" (Dubler, 1987, p. 147).

Protective services (Kapp, 1985) represent another intervention mechanism, one which has the potential of being less intrusive than either the guardianship or the conservatorship. "Protective service programs are characterized by two elements that can be mixed in an array of ways: the coordinated delivery of services to adults at risk, and the actual or potential authority to provide substitute decision-making" (Kapp and Bigot, 1985, p. 103). Although protective service statutes vary widely from state to state, the broad scope and flexibility, which are typical of the statutes, do have the advantage of allowing minimally intrusive interventions to be designed.

A somewhat more limited form of intervention is available in instances where financial self-neglect or mismanagement is alleged or evident. Representative payees may be appointed in cases where persons who regularly receive money from the government for pensions, disabilities, or other benefits are incapable of managing those funds themselves.

Finally, another form of intervention is the use of powers of attorney. The power of attorney represents a voluntary delegation of decision-making authority to another person, and it may be as broad or limited as the person delegating authority desires. The traditional power of attorney, however, has two principal limitations: at the time authority is delegated, the individual must be competent to make this authorization, and the authorization typically ceases if the individual becomes incapacitated (Kapp and Bigot, 1985, p. 108). In recognition of these problems, coming into more frequent use is the durable power of attorney. This device overcomes the problems associated with the power of attorney by specifying either that it is effective even if the individual becomes incapacitated or that it goes into effect when the person becomes incapacitated.

As we suggested above, these mechanisms represent a continuum of interventions, ranging from the most to the least restrictive and intrusive. They reflect maximum infringement upon autonomy at one extreme to minimal infringement at the other. Also, each is a legal mechanism, and many require judicial deliberation and determination. Fortunately, other forms of intervention — both formal and informal — exist. These include the broad array of formal community services, which can be provided to frail or self-neglecting elders, as well as the informal support systems of families, friends, and neighbors of older persons. Both sets of supportive assistance may be appropriately used when a determination has been made that beneficent intervention is warranted.

When a choice must be made among these various forms of intervention, it seems reasonable to suggest that the mechanism(s) should be carefully matched with the self-neglecting individual's condition and circumstances. Here, the principle of the least restrictive alternative (Dudovitz, 1985; Cohen, 1985) is applicable. In considering the range of possible interventions, professionals should always seek those that intrude to the least extent possible on a person's autonomy while simultaneously attempting to maximize the likelihood of attaining the desired protective outcome. It makes no sense to petition for the involuntary commitment of a self-neglecting elder if the provision of a homemaker or health aide will suffice to bring about the desired outcome. The critical challenge is to strike the right balance between preserving (and even enhancing) autonomy and protecting the self-neglecting individual through beneficent paternalism.

SUMMARY AND CONCLUSION

The purpose of this chapter has been to set forth the broad outlines of an ethical framework for use in considering cases of self-neglecting elders and for evaluating appropriate management options. We have attempted to establish the relevance of several major ethical principles — autonomy, beneficence, paternalism, and justice — which are often implicit in the deliberations of those who deal with self-neglect. By making these principles explicit, by illustrating their pertinence through case studies, and by noting how in actual situations they lend themselves to action guidelines, we hope to have demonstrated the value of ethical analysis.

As important as these ethical principles may be, we make no claim that their use will inevitably or easily lead professionals and practitioners to the answer in every case. Agreement about the proper or morally defensible course of action to take when confronting a self-neglecting elder is, as we have noted, likely to be reached more readily as situations approach the extremes. The lucid and competent elder whose self-neglecting behavior has minimal, if any, effect on others deserves to have his or her autonomous wishes and preferences respected. Just as clearly, intervention is the proper course of action when dealing with an impaired, incompetent elder whose self-neglect puts others at risk.

In many instances, however, the circumstances are not clear-cut, and the factual evidence upon which the ethical analysis must be based is less compelling: competence cannot be established decisively or the risk of harm cannot be determined precisely or the scales for weighing various costs and benefits are not equivalent. Furthermore, reasonable and well-meaning persons may bring different value systems to the situation of self-neglect, causing them to weigh principles differently and making it more difficult to reach agreement. Still, we would maintain that the systematic and structured application of ethical principles to cases of self-neglect will help to clarify underlying value differences, frame complex issues in a way that will promote productive discourse, and facilitate the process of arriving at a consensus about appropriate courses of action.

4

Psychiatric and Biomedical Considerations in Self-Neglect

Raymond Vickers

This chapter discusses psychiatric and biomedical aspects of self-neglect from the perspective of assessment. Whenever self-neglecting behavior is present, it is important to undertake a comprehensive evaluation. If possible, that assessment should be provided by an interdisciplinary team; however, core knowledge is needed to understand the extent to which psychiatric and medical conditions can be treated in order to help the elderly person attain the highest level of health and well-being. The focus of this discussion of clinical assessment covers cognitive and psychiatric disorders, biomedical conditions, and nutritional factors that have a direct and indirect impact on self-neglect and self-enhancement in old age. Models of interdisciplinary team assessment are reviewed as an appropriate strategy for evaluating cases of self-neglect.

SELF-NEGLECT AND MENTAL DISORDERS

There are many ways in which the will to survive, the mental processes that operationalize this will, and the personal capacities to carry out these processes may result in survival despite self-neglect. Evaluating the mental health of a self-neglecting elder may culminate in a judgment about the mental processes of survival and the extent to which distortion of these processes (so-called mental illness) might impair the capacity to survive. Optimally, mental health assessment should include an investigation of the effect of any complicating health condition that may contribute to self-neglect risks (Vickers, 1988). Inclusion of the medical component can make the task of assessment more demanding as the clinician tries to determine the role of primary mental illness in causing neglect, the effect of neglect on mental functioning, and the influence of the numerous biomedical conditions that may coexist (Rubenstein et al., 1989). This assessment process is performed particularly well by a multidisciplinary team, but even if a single clinician completes the assessment, the first task is recognition of those symptomatic patterns of primary psychiatric conditions most likely to be present in the older self-neglecting client.

Part of the mental health evaluation process is to describe the findings in diagnostic terms. In the United States, the current approved diagnostic terminology is based on the *Diagnostic and Statistical Manual of the American Psychiatric Association* (APA, 1987). The revised third edition of the DSM-III R manual calls for a rating on a series of so-called axes, which include a psychiatric diagnosis (Axis I), a personality classification (Axis II), a listing of significant medical conditions (Axis III), severity of psychosocial stressors (Axis IV), and global assessment of functioning (Axis V). Keeping in mind that ratings on these different axes provide the foundation for a psychiatric diagnosis, what follows is a brief review of those diagnostic categories likely to be applied in cases of self-neglect that are referred for evaluation to a community geriatric team (Vickers, 1976).

Transient adjustment reactions of later life (Adjustment Disorder) are those conditions strong enough to interfere with independent daily living but not permanent so as to constitute a psychiatric disability. The community's expectation that all people should be independent in performing activities of daily living (ADL) and instrumental activities of daily living (IADL) is deeply ingrained by the cultural attitudes about the maturation process. Thus, with the threat of lowered capacity in any of these activity areas, strong emotional reactions may occur, and the person experiencing the loss of ability can also have denial, anger, and grief. When these emotional symptoms become the principal reason for a mental health referral, the terms "transient situational personality disturbance" or "adjustment disorder of late life" are likely to be applied based on the assumption that if the symptoms continue they will be self-limiting.

These emotional states tend to be modified by psychological defense mechanisms, such as rationalization, projection, and reaction formation, resulting in the so-called psychoneurotic reactions of anxiety and depression. However, many older people do not seem to have the mental makeup that converts the painful emotional reactions to lost activity performance capacity into the relative shelter of neurotic defenses. They continue in denial, anger, or grief either because their narcissistic needs cannot accept an impaired self-image (MacLeod, 1988) or because of impaired cognitive capacity as is seen in some kinds of stroke (House and Hodges, 1988). Other individuals develop a dissociative reaction or psychotic depression and become totally helpless. These people may become unable to care for themselves and regress into severe states of self-neglect if appropriate and timely intervention is not provided.

In the aged, anxiety, depression, and suicidal feelings are the second most common group of psychological reactions. It has been estimated that 17 percent of older males and 22 percent of older females have a level of long-standing anxiety that needs treatment (Himmelfarb and Murrell, 1984), and about 15 percent to 20 percent of elderly patients living in the community have either a major depression or a significant degree of dysphoria (Blazer, 1989). It has been claimed that people who do not encounter medical stress until later life are likely to become depressed whereas those who have had earlier life medical problems are more likely to react with anxiety (Magni and De Leo, 1984). Often, anxiety is thought not to require psychiatric evaluation, perhaps because of the widespread use of minor tranquilizers (benzodiazepines) by primary physicians or the unjustified belief in the therapeutic value of reassurance. In the absence of treatment, many anxious elderly people slip into paranoid withdrawal or, in extreme cases, phobic hermitage.

Of patients referred for consultation to a geropsychiatric service (Vickers, 1976), more than one-third are anxious and clinically depressed, especially if the referrals include those who are medically ill or live in a long-term nursing facility. Elderly persons have difficulty in seeking help when they are depressed and find it hard to admit feeling sad or thinking about death. They are likely to have somatic conversions or preoccupations with an apparent symptom of serious physical illness such as heart disease (Davis-Berman, 1990; Gurland, 1976). Commonly seen is a state of depletion or disengagement known as helplessness-hopelessness syndrome (Solomon, 1990). Depression also appears in ambiguous forms. Many elderly show an agitated state, experience delusions (Meyers et al., 1984), or appear to have pseudodementia.

This last term is not a diagnostic condition included in the DSM-III R, but it is widely used to describe depressed patients who claim that their memory has been impaired. It is rare for a patient with actual organic dementia to complain of loss of memory, but there is usually some true memory loss in severe depression.

The diagnosis of depression in the elderly rests on either of two criteria. First, there may be a depressive syndrome present if a person scores positively on a depression scale designed for the elderly such as the Geriatric Depression Scale (Sheikh and Yesavage, 1986). The second criterion is the therapeutic response to treatment. Because more than 80 percent of depressed elderly, especially the more severe cases, improve with treatment, the diagnosis is confirmed by a response to therapy. In both classical depression and pseudodementia the association with self-neglect is often obvious as physical deprivation conditions are usually sufficiently severe and obvious to command immediate attention. Frequently these patients are convinced they are losing their minds, are seriously neglectful of activities of daily living, do not eat or sleep properly, and may be extremely reclusive because of shame and despair (Morris et al., 1989). When contacted with offers of assistance, they may express feeling unworthy of help and claim to want to die and be left alone.

In cases of severe agitation, the self-destructive element may be manifest and take the form of overt attempts at self-harm up to and including suicide. The possibility of suicide is always real among the elderly as their rate is more than double the average for all ages (McIntosh and Hubbard, 1988). Suicide should be anticipated in isolated older persons, and their attempts are more uniformly lethal than in younger age groups (Conwell et al., 1990). Because geriatric suicidal acts are so often completed, it is probably unjustified to use the term "suicidal equivalence" for cases of self-neglect, especially if combined with the belief that starvation might have been chosen by the victim as easier or more ethically acceptable than violent self-destruction (Simon, 1989).

Dementia is characterized by a cognitive defect of all higher intellectual capacity, caused by neuron loss (Thomas, 1989). The person who has a cognition deficit due to Alzheimer's disease or a related disorder will have a progressive loss of competence in self-care. Dementia-based cognitive loss has a much slower onset than that resulting from delirium or pseudodementia. This slow progressive deterioration may go undetected for a long period. By the time the demented individual is noticed, the effects of self-neglect, such as dangerous nutritional status or skin integrity, the presence of disease or of other public health dangers, may constitute an emergency. On occasion the best action to take in a crisis situation where the individual is isolated may be to initiate a temporary involuntary commitment. Isolation, however, is not a universal precondition for self-neglect to reach a life-threatening crisis. Some elderly people with slow progressive self-neglect behaviors continue to live in the presence of unheeding or irresolute families.

The diagnosis of dementia is based on a determination that there is a loss of cognitive function in more than one cerebral area, a significant degree of impairment as determined by mental status tests, and the exclusion of other mental syndromes. A few other syndromes must be excluded, especially those that are reversible with appropriate treatment, but 50 percent or more of cases of dementia are of the Alzheimer's type for which no specific drug treatment is available (Bartus, 1990). Many complications of the disease, such as self-neglect, however, can be ameliorated (Mace and Rabins, 1981).

Delirium, a potentially reversible disorder, is often undetected or misdiagnosed in the elderly. No other mental condition has a wider variety of causes, most of them medical rather than psychiatric (Lipowski, 1989). There is usually a disturbance of attention and consciousness, and when this appears in the form of acute confusion the person is often incapable of self-care. Other symptoms of delirium include stupor, agitation, hallucinations, and bizarre or frantic behavior. More subtle forms of quiet delirium occur with some frequency in elderly people and may be caused by vitamin-B deficiencies, electrolyte and other disturbances, and from cardiovascular drugs, chronic alcohol or sedative drug consumption, AIDS syndrome, and brain trauma. These are likely to be overlooked, and if self-neglecting behavior occurs the underlying cause may not be recognized because of the transitory nature of some of the symptoms.

Delirium is usually mistaken for dementia because both conditions are accompanied by loss of memory, delusions, and disorientation, but delirium has a relatively rapid onset and is likely to be accompanied by visual hallucinations and changes in the level of alertness. Unlike dementia, it is likely to become worse if small doses of tranquilizers are used. Sometimes the diagnosis can only be made retrospectively after symptoms abate, which is the pattern that differentiates it from dementia. The EEG is almost always abnormal in delirium but not in dementia. Many of the medical causes of delirium will result in permanent brain damage or death if they are not treated. Early recognition and treatment of delirium is necessary if the physical consequences of prolonged neglect are to be avoided (Tobias et al., 1989).

Paranoid reactions, commonly associated with some mental disorders in older people, may include severe withdrawal and self-neglecting behavior. Paranoia, the psychiatric syndrome in which the personality is intact except for severe delusions, often of persecution limited to one subject area, is rare in the elderly, but paranoid delusions are common. Paranoid symptoms appear for the first time in late life in 2 percent to 4 percent of aging persons, especially those who have suffered multiple losses. The symptoms seem to be an alternative expression to depression. The symptoms make it hard to help the affected individuals because of the high degree of suspiciousness that characterizes the condition. Often paranoid symptoms extend to food and drugs and cause rapid and visible self-neglect. Paranoid symptoms are often present among institutionalized self-neglecting elders who are engulfed by the well-meaning attention of staff, with the result being increased levels of patient anxiety.

Many street people with strange and unacceptable behaviors are labeled with the diagnosis of chronic schizophrenia. Where they have a long history of schizophrenic symptomatology, especially if it required their prolonged stay in a psychiatric institution, this may be valid. The policies of release, which replaced that of institutionalization, have sent numbers of such symptomatic individuals into the community, especially in certain areas. They are often socially unprepared and constitutionally unfit to live a healthy, independent existence and become victims of self-neglect, if not overt abuse. However, this is a disease primarily of the first half of the life span, and many recover with treatment, so it is not at all common in the elderly. Of those who become chronic, the positive symptoms often ameliorate, and the negative ones tend to improve. Many of these people function very well with maintenance psychotropic drugs; the discontinuance of these drugs may produce the most obvious cases of deterioration and neglect (Cohen et al., 1988).

Alcoholism and other substance abuse affects as many as 10 percent of the community elderly (Gomberg and Lisansky, 1988). The elderly alcoholic who survives tends to keep a balance between the daily alcohol intake and its desired effects. Those who cannot achieve this equilibrium usually do not survive into old age. The primary self-neglect symptoms are often not those of drunkenness, but of falls, hypothermia, malnutrition, and neglect of personal hygiene. These symptoms are often misdiagnosed as indicators of dementia. All aspects of self-care, both primary and instrumental activities of daily living, are likely to be neglected by aged persons in active states of severe alcoholism. In a sense, consumption of alcohol and drugs are symptoms of self-neglect rather than causes. If the goal of treatment is substantial improvement of the functioning of the elderly alcoholic, it is essential to consider the reason for the substance abuse (Benshoff and Robberto, 1987).

Personality disorder is a term often used to describe many individuals suffering from self-neglect. It is important to differentiate personality traits, common to all people throughout the life span, from personality disorders, which may cause serious problems in daily living. Patients with antisocial and histrionic personality disorder may defy the usual social expectations for self-care or present a narcissistic haughtiness toward persons attempting to help. These individuals are very difficult to help because they systematically refuse to cooperate with potential care providers. As a consequence they may suffer from serious neglect. Some elders respond to offers of help by acting out their unconscious wishes or conflicts, and their aggressive or seductive behaviors can become unmanageable. Persons with dependent personality disorder may overwhelm the service provider with insatiable demands. Hypochondriacal and borderline per-sonalities are dissatisfied with almost any effort on their behalf and maintain a reproachful attitude toward those offering help. Individuals with passive-aggressive responses, such as procrastination and self-harm, may be among those at greatest risk of self-neglect. Any of the above behaviors may constitute a "cry for help" among some elderly people or present as "pseudo-independent dependency" (Goldfarb, 1969).

Elderly persons with these disorders are often referred to psychiatric staff after numerous community care providers have exhausted their repertoire of available services. They may be described in the referral record as "acting-out," which is often misused as a wastebasket designation for all resistive behavior (Aronson et al., 1983). These behaviors provoke referrals of the "troublemakers" to the police for punishment or to hospitals for confinement. Neither law enforcement nor acute general hospital staff are usually well equipped to manage the behavioral problems that lead to the labels and efforts to control the disruptors. Few strategies may be available to deal with the arrested or ostracized person. Tranquilizers, often used even forcibly to settle these individuals into compliant modes, only serve to convert one problem into another and rarely provide anything but a short-term sedation of the patient.

There are several important basic steps for the clinician trying to assess the person's presenting condition. The first is to offer a reasonable diagnosis based on as accurate and extensive information as can be gathered under crisis-like conditions. The next step is to identify someone who can communicate with the individual, who despite the aggressive mannerism is often alone and afraid. A trusted intermediary can often facilitate the clinician's communication with the patient by virtue of reducing the clinician's image as the total authority figure. Under conditions such as these, treatment contracts may have no impact on controlling the behavior of the client, if that is the intent of such agreements. Waiting to negotiate the process of offering help and having it rejected until the client can accept that his welfare might improve may be more compatible with an individual's rights and ultimate welfare than forcing treatment onto the unwilling person (Kapp, 1988).

Clinical staff can work with these individuals for a long time without making any progress toward their engagement. An illustration of one case may help to clarify the challenge of establishing a working alliance with the client.

An elderly street woman was reported by the press to be camping out in freezing weather in a packing box across from City Hall. The media were quick to expose the authorities' "neglect" of this former mental patient. When the mental health worker told her that an adequate residential shelter was available, she refused to use the facility. The community response was to suggest commitment to a state hospital as the solution. Finally, against the protest of the mental health worker, the police solved the problem by deporting her to a warm southern state. She was last heard of when the Atlanta news media discovered her living in a packing box under an overpass at the junction of two busy streets.

In this case the community was pressing to get the mental health authorities to provide the quick solution by first offering the option of a shelter bed and then progressing to order her into an inpatient situation when she refused the first option. Her personality disorder did not equate to mental incompetence even though the community viewed her behavior as bizarre and her presence as an eyesore. The pressure to get her out of the way precluded the worker from having the opportunity to establish a relationship with her and/or to identify someone from her network who could help explore acceptable alternatives.

Unlike long-term personality disorders, organic personality syndrome may have a late life onset, and it may accompany epilepsy or result from head injury. One form of the syndrome produces apathy with gross indifference to self-care without regard to danger or self-exposure. Another form involves emotional lability with episodes of crying or unpredictable anger and assaultiveness. These behaviors make the individual a very unwelcome resident in shelters that are understaffed or in facilities that have neither the space nor the staff resources to manage difficult patients. Sometimes these individuals are most welcome on the streets by other people already established in the street culture, who accept them and provide some sense of safe comradeship.

Patterns of depressive and self-destructive behaviors can result from focal neurological damage to the brain (Orrell et al., 1989). This damage can result from the readily recognizable acute vascular stroke or from less commonplace injuries, tumors, or epileptic conditions, which require skilled diagnoses (Robinson et al., 1984). One of the most complex of these conditions is the hemicorporeal neglect syndrome, which occurs with nondominant parietal strokes in which the person is no longer aware of the affected half of the body. Injury or other forms of endangering neglect may occur because of an organic-based denial by the affected person (Mark and Heilman, 1990). Although the community-based worker does not have the responsibility of differentiating between these various syndromes, it is important to know that they might exist. Being able to arrange for an adequate neuropsychological examination to confirm a suspected brain-damaged person may be a miraculous feat, given the lack of space to diagnose those without insurance.

Older individuals with bipolar affective disorders, previously termed "manic-depressive reactions," are less likely to experience hyperactive behavior than middle-aged persons who enter a manic phase. The diagnosis is often missed in older patients, but the characteristic self-neglect is usually present in both the manic and depressive phases. One of the systemic problems contributing to improper diagnosis is the shuttling of patients back and forth from setting to setting, making it impossible to formulate a longitudinal picture of the patterns of manic-to-depressive-to-manic shifts. Lithium has been reported to have a positive impact on improving the patient's functional capacity for self-care, but the improvement can be lost if medication is discontinued (Rubin, 1988).

Until recently, mental retardation was not compatible with survival until late life. Better medical care has prolonged the life expectation of many retarded people, who after significant periods of institutionalization are now living their later years in community settings. Because of the long periods of institutional care, many of these older adults were socialized into high levels of dependence. This pattern can be successfully reversed with community-oriented social skills training provided by a skilled specialist. With careful planning, this group of potentially self-neglecting older people can be successful in community living and social participation within the aging service network (Seltzer et al., 1989).

This abbreviated discussion of the interconnections between geriatric psychiatric conditions that are known to have numerous and diverse impacts on the behavioral problem of self-neglect is intended as a general orientation to one of the two fundamental components of assessment. The other dimension of assessment must encompass the evaluation of biomedical conditions. In the elderly, knowledge of biomedical status very often proves to be the key to providing interventions that eliminate or at least reduce self-neglect and associated risks.

BIOMEDICAL CONDITIONS AFFECTING BEHAVIOR

The concept of basic needs is useful in this context because the biomedical assessment of problems of self-neglecting elders always touches on quality-of-life issues and frequently involves confronting patient problems that may threaten survival. Maslow (1954) points out that humans tend to prioritize their basic needs and fulfill the most primal physiological ones first before progressing to meet other needs according to a general hierarchy. When an elderly person cannot meet the physiological needs essential to survival, the baseline of life is diminished and must become the first treatment goal of medical care. Using a biological processes framework, the author discusses what he considers relevant in order to attain a holistic view of assessment among aged persons suspected of self-neglect.

Basic needs, if met, support three fundamental internal biological processes essential for life:

1. Anabolism is the process resulting in the metabolic outcomes of growth, storage, and repair. The basic external needs are nutrition, water, and oxygen; there are also secondary internal needs for digestion, storage, respiration, and circulation.
2. Catabolism is the process providing for the release of energy from some of the consumed food or the supplies of fat and glycogen stored by anabolism, with the production of breakdown products. The energy is used in movement or is reutilized by anabolism with the production of heat. An excretory system is required to eliminate waste breakdown products.
3. Reactivity is a process meeting the need for stimulation, or informational flow from the environment and its storage, the need for activity (a high-reactive state responding to both internal and external stimuli), and the need for rest (a low-reactive state mostly responding to internal stimuli). Internally these functions are all sustained by the nervous system through its sensory, cognitive, autonomic, and motor components and by neuroendocrine secretion. Reactivity also serves as a mechanism to regulate the rate of anabolism and catabolism, producing a complex but homeostatically balanced organism (Dilman, 1981).

Disturbance in the supply of external needs, or the ability of the body to continue these internal processes, will constitute a hazard to the individual. The primary task in performing a biomedical evaluation of a self-neglecting individual is to attempt to detect and measure such changes in the supply of external needs to sustain internal processes. Assessment gives attention to the sources available to the individual to provide supplies whereby the internal processes can occur, and consider how the result of deprivation and disease interfere.

The elderly experience numerous internal problems that may prevent sufficient oxygen from reaching the brain; therefore, medical evaluation needs to measure the adequacy of its amount and flow. Strangulation of the downward air flow into the lungs during sleep is a condition affecting many elderly patients. Sleep-disordered breathing in which snoring is accompanied by many periods of apnea, periods of absent respirations each hour, is now considered a significant geriatric problem and may contribute to subsequent heart damage, hypertension, and mental illness due to brain damage from hypoxia, a decreased saturation of the blood with oxygen (Morewitz, 1988). Compensatory daytime somnolence can also be implicated in self-neglect.

Difficulty in breathing due to obstructive changes in the lower airways of the lungs is another area of concern. Puffing and blowing are often blamed on old age despite the fact that such difficulties are found almost exclusively in cigarette smokers. Chronic bronchitis, another type of obstruction, is accompanied by coughing and wheezing due to an increase in sputum from the thickened mucous lining of the airways. Emphysema is caused by a reduction in the number of alveoli needed for adequate oxygen absorption into the blood, which results in progressive shortness of breath.

Chronic bronchitis and emphysema are found together and may be associated with asthma. These conditions constitute the complex known as Chronic Obstructive Lung Disease (COPD), which disables large numbers of the elderly by decreasing their exercise capacity (Reichel, 1989). Decreased exercise levels may go unnoticed because it is easy for people to adjust their effort level downward as they grow older, and the extent of initial loss is only likely to show at times of peak physical exertion. Affected people are forced to do less for themselves and ultimately neglect even the most essential tasks of daily living. Partial relief may be obtained from using aerosol spray inhalers, but advanced COPD is resistant to treatment, especially in those who continue smoking and ultimately compromise oxygenation and, therefore, brain function. Heavy smoking can be interpreted as another manifestation of self-neglect. An additional factor to be considered is that there may be personality changes secondary to the drugs commonly used for asthma such as prednisone, sympathomimetics, and atropine analogs, all of which can cause organic hallucinosis and paranoid states.

The oxygen transport capacity of the blood is a product of the hemoglobin in the red blood cells. Anemia, which results from a lack of hemoglobin, initially causes an increased circulatory output to make up for the decreased capacity. Later the chronic presence of anemia slows down the whole body metabolism, causing the individual to become languorous and easily exhausted, which can contribute to self-neglect. Conversely, even though acute failure of the circulation results in immediate oxygen lack in the tissues, light-headedness, and even coma, it is chronic heart failure that produces the extreme lassitude that can result in neglect.

When conducting a medical assessment, particularly when doing it in a community setting, few technological or personnel supports may be available. Even so, questions must be asked of the elderly person to determine any history of shortness of breath, cough and sputum, the loss of blood, chest pain, palpitation, or evidence of fever, history of tuberculosis, or AIDS exposure. Additional information about nutritional status is important because it has great influence on the ability of the lungs to protect against infection. The portion of the physical examination to evaluate respiratory function should observe whether there is dyspnea and if it is present when the individual is stationary or at any point of exertion, as well as if cyanosis is present.

The alternation of periods of active movement and adequate rest constitutes a vital need and may become a challenge to successful aging. There are many myths about sleep in old age, and although aging brings some changes in sleep patterns, it is sleep deprivation that can be most harmful to physical and psychological functioning (Burnside, 1988). It is a cause for physical depletion and mood change and can lead to disorientation that reinforces other self-neglecting tendencies.

Exercise is recognized as an essential aspect of healthy aging. Many cases of self-neglect occur because of activity restriction due to skeletal, muscle, and joint conditions as well as many other kinds of pain. Real and fantasied dangers keep many older people in great exercise privation. The difficulty of movement or the intentional failure to move may be connected to psychoenvironmental conditions that contribute to some self-neglect. For example, an elderly person's fear of falling may be the primary factor in avoiding food preparation, or fear of opening the front door because of crime may be so great as to prevent someone from taking advantage of home delivered food, with malnutrition as a direct result.

Deficits in the nervous system influence psychological and neurological control of the body and the capacity to satisfy basic biophysical needs. The reactivity process is initially dependent on sensory input from the environment especially through sound and vision. Visual effects of uncorrected refractive errors, undetected glaucoma, unrelieved cataracts, and unremitting macular degeneration are some of the more prevalent barriers to information retrieval that affect mobility. Hearing impairment also causes information deficit through such basic experiences as conversation. If communication is distorted, there is a barrier to a routine source of knowledge about the world around us, as well as to warnings of immediate danger (Corso, 1981). As mentioned earlier, the reactivity process can also be hampered by the effects of strokes, dementia, and psychosis impacting on information storage and processing. In cases of self-neglect, the clinician's assessment of these biomedical conditions should help to restore or strengthen the elder's reactivity process so as to aid sensory connections to the environment.

The neuroendocrine system consists of the internal secretion glands and the parts of the neurological system that control the rate of anabolism and catabolism. There seems to be a marked variation in the capacity of the aging thyroid, adrenal, and pancreas glands to react to a stress demand for increased secretion. Even though estimates of endocrine functioning are imprecise, these conditions are worth investigating in the assessment process. Because an estimated 15 percent of elderly persons have diabetes, a glucose test is an important screening procedure in this process. Lowered thyroid function is often not recognized in the 4 percent of the elderly in which it occurs, yet it may result in the slowing of body systems and, as a consequence, self-neglect. A person with untreated myxedema shows evidence of premature aging and should be correctly identified (Zellman, 1978). So-called apathetic hyperthyroidism in the elderly is also a cause of marked self-neglect and requires a screening blood test for diagnosis (Helford and Crapo, 1990). Loss of function of the adrenal glands (Addison's disease) results in a gradual increase in lethargy, weakness, and mental symptoms such as irritability and delusions. The skin may become bronzed in color, and tuberculosis or AIDS may coexist (Bondy, 1985).

The task of excretion, which characterizes catabolism, requires the removal of numerous chemicals including acid through the lungs (carbon dioxide) and kidneys, nitrogen and poisons through the kidneys, and food wastes from the bowel. With all of these types of excretion, limited quantities of water are also extracted. Paradoxically, many of the same diseases that cause obstruction of bowel and bladder may also cause incontinence. Incontinence, a physical condition with social ramifications, may affect as many as 30 percent of the community aged (Diokno et al., 1986). Breakdown of the social network may follow the development of incontinence because of social unacceptability. It is essential for those who work with the elderly to recognize this association and accept the fact that clinicians will need the proper attitude and skills to cope with incontinence as part of geriatric practice (Baigis-Smith et al., 1989).

NUTRITIONAL ASPECTS OF NEGLECT

There is widespread concern about the nutrition of the nation's aged. The growth of the federally sponsored Nutritional Program for Older Americans (Older Americans Act, Title III) has provided for nutritional supplementation and minimal dietary counseling to millions of older people. However, that program is sometimes not available in the home, so many homebound cannot benefit. Nevertheless, some politicians claim that with the program, malnutrition is no longer a problem. Political optimism and/or widespread lack of medical concern about the importance of diet may be blocking further attention to national strategies to improve nutrition in late life. The Medicare program (Social Security Act, Title XVIII) does not include payment for ambulatory and home care nutritional services even in cases of diabetes and heart disease, which have major dietary implications.

Nutrient deficiencies are important, both as a consequence and, occasionally, as a cause of self-neglect in the elderly, because there is some evidence that a lack of water-soluble vitamins contributes to mental impairment (Goodwin et al., 1983). As a by-product, elderly individuals who suffer from malnutrition may be mistakenly diagnosed with dementia. The author recommends that the assessment of biomedical needs for all individuals suspected of self-neglect include evaluation of the diet, symptoms of specific nutritional deficiencies, and, wherever possible, interpretation of laboratory tests (Morley, 1986).

Feeding Problems

Anorexia is a problem with many possible causes. There may have been a lifelong habitual pattern of difficulties in eating, due to a shortage of food, a lack of appetite, a willful refusal to eat, or a mechanical difficulty in taking food in, chewing or swallowing it. Beliefs about food are often acquired at an early age and held tenaciously throughout life. When social isolation and physical changes, such as the loss of teeth, disrupt eating patterns, adaptation may not occur, and nutritional deprivation results. Sometimes, voluntary refusal to eat is a real way for a person to express unwillingness to go on living, and this is the basis of some cases of self-neglect. If a good nutritional history is available, one may discover a pattern of hunger strikes in earlier life when such an individual could not resolve difficult situations. With age, intentional fasting may become dangerous. Failure to eat as an expression of loss of hope may be precipitated by the real or fanciful discovery of a disease that the individual dreads. It may not be the dramatic illnesses that are most feared, but physical disability, impotency, blindness, or deafness, which looms as a potential loss of independence. It is known that deafness is more frequently associated with isolation and suicidal acts than blindness; this may mean that loss of significant communication is feared most of all possible losses.

Certain psychiatric conditions are characterized by poor eating. Schizophrenia, paranoid disorders, and depression are all conditions in which severe malnutrition as well as other aspects of self-neglect can be seen.

Alzheimer's disease is usually accompanied by poor eating habits, and loss of weight may be the presenting symptom. People with advanced cases of this and other dementias may have difficulty in remembering that they are eating long enough to finish a meal, yet they often report feeling hungry immediately after eating. It has been suggested that because the earliest signs of Alzheimer's disease are found in the hippocampus, directly connected with the organ of smell through the first cranial nerve, gustatory loss may be a casualty of the first neurons damaged by the disease. Because the aroma of food is lost, the appetite is not stimulated. People with dementia may also have difficulty in swallowing because of lack of reactivity to the presence of food in their mouth.

Dysphagia, difficulty in swallowing, is caused by many neurological conditions, such as stroke, and certain psychotropic medications, such as major tranquilizers, as well as alcohol.

Aspiration of food or liquids is a serious threat. It may cause bronchitis or pneumonia and can result in asphyxia and death. Patients surviving this experience are often very fearful of eating. Additionally, many neurological disorders result in tremor, weakness, and paralysis, and this affects all aspects of self-care including obtaining food and maintaining its hygiene and safety in storage, cooking, and waste disposal. Often the skills of eating are lost or made so difficult that the person is frustrated and discouraged from feeding adequately.

Lassitude and fatigue from chronic illness often contribute to poor food intake and self-neglect. Cancer, one of the most common causes of mortality, is the first condition that comes to mind when weakness and loss of weight are found, particularly when other causes cannot be identified. The catabolic potential of cancer as a wasting disease is frequently compounded by severe anorexia. Coronary heart disease and heart failure, the other most frequent causes of death in the elderly, may involve many years of weakness, pain (often thought to be indigestion), and a sensation of impending death. These may also cause illnesses resulting from failure to eat adequately. Liver failure, especially in alcoholics, causes loss of appetite and is accompanied by protein-vitamin deficiencies, as are most other gastrointestinal disorders. Diabetes, a widespread metabolic disease of the elderly, results in catabolic wasting; it may affect appetite adversely and may also cause difficulty in swallowing. Chronic infections such as AIDS, tuberculosis, and urinary tract sepsis are significant causes of both anorexia and increased catabolism (Marton et al., 1981).

Toxicity, most commonly found in old people as a result of medications use and misuse (both over-the-counter and prescribed), is a potent cause of poor nutrition. A careful drug history is an essential part of the nutritional assessment because the anorexic effect of medication is often overlooked. For instance, digoxin (a form of digitalis) is one of the most commonly prescribed cardiac medications in the elderly, but it is likely to cause serious anorexia, which may result in nutritional deficiency. Many other drugs, including widely advertised antiarthritis medications, potassium supplements, and chemotherapy, cause loss of appetite and have other toxic effects, but the most common poison ingested by humans continues to be alcohol. Chronic alcohol consumption can lead to malnutrition because the gastritis it produces destroys the appetite; malabsorption of fats, zinc, and B-vitamins occur; and functions of the liver, heart, bone marrow, and brain may be damaged. Antacids reduce absorption of total calories, thiamine, and folic acid. Laxatives interfere with absorption of B2 and B12, fat-soluble vitamins, and calcium. Salicylates can interfere with vitamin C intake, and vitamin C can reduce B12 absorption. A careful drug history is a critical element in any nutritional assessment even though it is often difficult to quantify past and present medication compliance.

Protein-Calorie Malnutrition

Malnutrition affected by protein-calorie balance will ultimately result from inadequate food intake if the body's supply is exhausted from starvation or anorexia. The risk of this type of malnutrition is greatest among the impoverished elderly. Despite general perceptions, not all malnourished individuals are underweight. Obesity can be a type of malnourishment if it results from a high starch diet poor in protein (Kohrs et al., 1979).

Protein and zinc deficiency seem to cause a loss of taste and smell, which are connected to appetite and food enjoyment. Protein deficiency causes anorexia and diarrhea. As a result, once a deficiency has been established, food intake may become progressively reduced and malabsorption increased. Certain vitamin and mineral deficiencies commonly accompany protein deficiency, because the main protein sources, meat and high-grade cereals, contain significant supplies of both. Thinning of the skin, loss of hair, edema of the extremities, increased susceptibility to disease, and failure of wounds to heal are all signs of protein and zinc insufficiency and contribute to chronic sores of the legs and feet in neglected individuals.

Vitamin deficiency can cause a wide variety of dermatological changes. Red scaly rash and sores can result from vitamin A, B, and C deficiencies, and hemorrhages from scurvy can be visible in the skin. Scurvy also causes bone pain, as does vitamin D deficiency. Prominent among potential deficiencies is the vitamin B group. Thiamine (B1), riboflavin (B2), niacin, pyridoxine (B6), vitamin B12, and folic acid are commonly lacking in the diet of elderly individuals. This may be the case among the poor who do not have the resources to purchase foods that are rich in B-vitamin. Symptoms of B-vitamin deficiency include sore mouth and mental confusion, both of which tend to perpetuate the condition.

Mineral disturbance may be life threatening in the elderly. Hyponatremia, or low-salt syndrome, is the most common type of mineral disturbance in the institutional setting where many patients receive diuretic drugs while they are also placed on low-salt diets. In contrast, hyponatremia is rarely seen in community-based elders who have not been under medical treatment. In unusual cases, long-term treatment with phenothiazine tranquilizers or the presence of head injury may produce this condition. Malnutrition can also produce a hyponatremia that is characterized by a serious lassitude leading to further self-neglect (Rose, 1989). Potassium, a mineral typically found in fruit, is significantly lacking in many diets. Older women, for whom exchangeable stores of potassium are already reduced, are most likely to show the effects of a low blood potassium (starvation hypokalemia). In addition to sodium and potassium, many other important minerals, including iron and calcium, are likely to be deficient in the chronically malnourished individual.

Water is an important component of good nutrition. As the body ages, reserves of water are reduced, making the individual more vulnerable to fluid imbalance. Many older people believe in the importance of drinking adequate quantities of water, but circumstances may arise when this belief is thwarted by their own incontinence or mobility problems or by caregivers frustrated by constant requests for fluids. For instance, one occasionally finds an incontinent person who is being secretly deprived of fluids in an effort to reduce urine output. Water deprivation is one of the most common results of neglect in institutions; patients may be given drinks only when meals are served or if they ask. An individual living alone with mobility problems may have problems reaching accessible water in the household.

A diminished sensation of thirst seems to occur with age, but it is especially noticeable when mental symptoms are present, as in dementia. Because caregivers are used to experiencing thirst whenever they need additional liquids, it is difficult for them to appreciate that an aged person may be in need of water and not request it. Older people will often not feel thirst when very dehydrated and may even refuse the fluids they need. If adequate water intake is not maintained, mental confusion may occur.

REFERRAL AND ASSESSMENT FOR SELF-NEGLECT PROBLEMS

Knowledge that mental health practitioners have about self-neglect may be essential for evaluating the needs and problems of elderly clients who are at risk. Psychiatrists usually participate in assessment based on some consultative arrangement with public agencies, a court-ordered mandate for completing a psychiatric diagnosis, and/or — in a smaller number of cases — as staff of a program attached to a mental health center where aged individuals have been referred as patients. The referral, whether mandated or voluntary, is usually the first step for linking elderly persons to a psychiatric resource. The content of the referral typically states that the elderly person is in desperate circumstances and that there is community concern about the dangers of self-neglect that pose a problem of personal or public safety. When danger to the person is the expressed concern, the usual focus is the risk of fire or injury rather than the effects of chronic self-neglect.

Phrasing the concern in terms of a threat to the individual or community complies with state and local statutes that protect the individual from interference based solely on lifestyle and residential maintenance. An example of this type of concern is reflected in the case of Mrs. W, an 81-year-old woman living with a menagerie of pets in a home full of junk. Piles of old newspapers, clothing, and other potentially flammable materials were found in every room. Those making the home visit had to assist each other across the mountains of junk. She was moderately impaired in mobility and had a fear of emerging into the outside community. The self-neglect was clear, but the justification for referral was stated in terms of her personal threats from the living condition rather than in relation to other consequences of her self-neglect.

Frequently, the person being evaluated is living alone or does not have visiting family. Less usually, neglecting individuals live with their families, and the whole interpenetration of family dynamics serves to complicate the assessment. In many cases, the family is the first and last source of help for the self-neglecting elder, and providing aid is regarded by some as an unquestionable duty. Moreover, referral to the formal support network is often delayed until family resources are quite exhausted. An informal support network of neighbors and old friends often supplements the efforts of the family, and the ultimate need for formal intervention may be regarded with shame by the recipient and guilt by the family and friends.

Assuming that a team format is used for the evaluation, it is important for team members conducting the assessment to appreciate the feelings of people in the informal network, because they influence the information offered about the elderly person (Brown et al., 1990). Well-meaning helpers may have fostered overdependency and may give the impression of greater need than is justified, or they may gloss over what they regard as embarrassing incompetency to save the dignity of the subject. Frequently the guilt that is generated by helpers' inability to cope is expressed as irritability and criticism of the worker. The evaluation of family stress is part of such an interview and may be completed through informal conversations, open-ended interviews, or through structured assessment tools.

A family tends to overemphasize certain dangers, such as the possibility that falls and strokes could leave a person maimed and unable to summon help. This position is reflected in such statements as, "I worry that I will not be there when Mother needs me." Families traditionally underemphasize other things, such as evidence the client might kill himself or the quantity of alcohol regularly consumed. They may be ambivalent about evidence of memory loss.

Complicating this situation are the psychosocial characteristics of the caregivers who may have needs to care for or to withhold care from others as part of their personality or because of some other need to control the elder. An example might be the man who cares for his elderly invalid wife but allows her to bathe without his assistance, although it is dangerous for her, because he is too uncomfortable to assist with her personal hygiene.

A particularly misleading area for discussion with relatives is that of institutionalization. This subject is so fraught with misinformation for the average member of the public, sometimes for professionals as well, that the worker must attempt a mini-education on the subject. Many families believe that mental health professionals conducting a psychiatric assessment in the home have the power to dispatch the client into an institutional setting. For the average family member not familiar with the laws protecting the elder's rights against forced institutionalization, talking about memory deficits is perceived as giving away a secret to justify a mental commitment. The reverse pattern may also operate where families are intentionally emphasizing the person's incompetence in hope that a removal from the current situation will be initiated by the mental health worker. The topic of a possible nursing home placement is also surrounded by guilt and fear, and quick decisions should be avoided in order to complete a full assessment and consider less restrictive options. Time is required to reach a new homeostasis for each person involved if there is to be some true give and take about a major change in the elder's residence.

Often when families request a mental health evaluation, it is because of some disturbance in domestic tranquility. A self-neglecting parent or spouse triggers family action and reaction. These family efforts may be rejected by the elder who withdraws from the family assistance that is needed for functioning. By the time the evaluation takes place, there is no evidence that any negotiations can produce an alternative to the alienation among family members. Sometimes, however, in the face of family conflict involving the elder's primary caregiver, it is useful to suggest respite as a less restrictive alternative that will prevent the angry family members from attempting to force some sort of inappropriate institutionalization.

Of the families who seek assessment, a minority stand to benefit financially from a finding of mental incompetence. The assessment team members should regard this as possible when there are material resources to control, although this is more often a subject for fiction than fact. Covetousness is directed not only at the rich; it is also possible when the resources are slim; purloining a Social Security check by a caregiver is not all that unusual. Under optimal circumstances, a community-based assessment should be undertaken only to assess the elderly person's functional condition.

Finally, the assessment team has the responsibility to recognize and interpret assumptions made by the family and others about the need for support based on traditional sex role stereotyping. On the one hand, the traditional role of the woman in the home may lead to a false sense of assurance that self-neglect is not taking place because it is unthinkable in a formerly competent housewife. Or, adult children may not believe that an aged father should do domestic work even if his not performing the tasks creates many risks. On the other hand, there is often undue haste to assume an aged man is self-neglecting simply because he has been waited on all of his life and is now alone. It is just as sexist to assume that all men need women to do the housework as it is to assume all women cannot maintain the financial accounts of the household. These stereotypes may be operating in the informal system and may create a source of resistance to suggestions that elderly persons complete tasks not associated with what is the traditional role. Age-sex role stereotyping is also a danger among professionals who interject these into their care planning.

The evaluating professional needs to be familiar with the various aspects of powers of attorney, custodianship, and conservatorship (see Chapters 3 and 10) so that observations made during the assessment process can provide accurate information for court decisions to limit the rights and the freedoms of the aged person. The importance of recording all observations and conclusions at the time of assessment cannot be overemphasized because such notes may be relevant to court decisions. To some extent, an already suspicious elder is not calmed by a worker who makes notes of everything, fearing the potential use of the information. A practitioner is responsible for explaining why he is recording during the assessment interview and to be honest about when, where, and how the information could be used.

CLIENT RESISTANCE TO ASSESSMENT

Many elderly people resist assessment. Although the mental health worker is not usually responsible for obtaining the elder's initial agreement for an assessment, the approach taken by the team at the time of the interview can increase or decrease client cooperation. Less cooperation is usually evidence of fear and misunderstanding. The experienced clinician who has done assessments in different settings, such as streets or shelters, knows the common response of a psychotic or paranoid person. Preparation for such reactions among elderly homebound persons is equally important. If there is reason to believe that an elderly person will be less threatened if a trusted person is present during the interview, then that person's presence and participation should be sought. These confidants can also be a good resource for future cooperation with the team if approached in a respectful way as a key person in a position to help the elderly individual.

The assessment should be offered to the elder as a gesture of help. Fear and resistance can sometimes be lessened if the elder knows that assessment is the necessary step to tap into a bureaucracy that controls helpful resources. It is difficult to minimize some of the legalistic and pater-nalistic conditions that surround many aspects of mandated assessment. The situational context for conducting the interview should, whenever possible, keep the elder's dignity as an ever present goal before, during, and after the assessment.

Assessment ordered by the courts typically requires some concrete diagnostic determination based on a measurable level of functional deficit as presented by the elder's behavior. The elder can display resistance by refusing to converse with the interviewers or by striving to convince the evaluator of independence. In circumstances such as these, finding reliable informants, having multiple visits, and reviewing data available from other professionals who know the client can improve the accuracy and comprehensiveness of assessment.

Community resources may be overlooked when assessing social supports because court authorization specifies that a psychiatric diagnosis is the single outcome of a mandated assessment, those completing the assessment have very limited knowledge of community resources (Rubenstein, 1987), or service resources known to team members are never easily accessed, so they are not suggested or pursued by staff.

The once popular use of involuntary hospital commitment sought in an emergency is no longer readily available or — in some states — actually illegal. The loss of this option is sometimes problematic because it prevents the team from gathering the biomedical information components previously described as vital to a mental health assessment. However, increasingly data suggest that assessments directed toward involuntary commitments have a poor reliability for predicting dangerousness to others (McNiel and Binder, 1987); it is probable that their ability to assess dangers to self are no more reliable.

To counter the pressure to institutionalize, mental health workers must be prepared to make varied types of assessment in the community (Herst, 1983). Not only do the bureaucratic agency requirements often limit the potential value and comprehensiveness of the in-home assessment, but also clinicians may feel incompetent to do assessment away from a controlled clinic environment and so do not make every effort to perform the assessment in the client's natural environment.

The single-shot assessment approach is not usually the best way to approach the determination of individual competency. To be competent one must have the capacity to reach a decision about not accepting help and the freedom to make the decision about help as well as full information about the likely consequences of the decision and the alternatives available. People who reject interventions may have a legal and ethical right to do so, but in doing so they often invite the assumption that they are mentally incompetent. They, therefore, often find themselves having to prove their competence to the larger community before they will find their right to refuse intervention honored.

THE MULTIDISCIPLINARY TEAM APPROACH: THE ALBANY MODEL

Primary care medical practitioners, public health nurses, and protective service workers are most likely to be the first professionals to see self-neglecting elders; they often make the initial evaluation. However, the best assessments are made by a multidisciplinary team (Campbell and Cole, 1987). The use of multidisciplinary resources during assessment has proved to be an effective way to match services to need, but this requires in turn that the mental health clinic has actually developed a mobile interdisciplinary geriatric team or its equivalent.

One of the earliest examples of the effectiveness of community outreach and multidisciplinary intervention for the elderly patient is the Capital District Psychiatric Center's Mobile Geriatric Screening Team organized in 1968 at Albany, New York. The unit was established as part of a program to find alternatives to admitting older persons to the regional state mental hospital (Markson et al., 1971). The team consisted of a psychiatrist, a psychologist, an internist, social workers, and psychiatric nurses. Referrals were seen in their natural surroundings by two or three workers and were reviewed at an interdisciplinary meeting the same or next day. Team members came to recognize the tremendous amount of information that would be obtained in a home visit, a fact now widely recognized in geriatric mental health (Ramsdell et al., 1989).

Community assessments conducted in the natural environment allow for an understanding of the related stressors and supports and direct professionals to tap the informal network of neighbors and friends. The Mobile Geriatric Team at Albany developed the practice of inviting as many of the informal support network as were available to participate in interviews. Their input offered a natural progression to the psychosocial history and behavioral changes, and the various points of view about the client's needs were easier to interpret in some logical and meaningful way. The involvement of these additional persons provided the information and the time to formulate a well-conceived treatment plan.

At first, the team saw only patients who had been referred for a decision about hospitalization. Many of these cases involved elderly persons suffering from the consequences of self-neglect. Sometimes this was associated with recognizable mental illness, but often it was not attributable to a psychiatric disorder. Following comprehensive assessment, the team recommended interventions of various kinds. They initiated steps for much needed medical care and detected and took action to reduce polypharmacy problems as well as activities of daily living deficits, such as those associated with malnutrition.

It soon became clear to the team that the most frequent cause of referral was depressive reaction, not dementia, as had been supposed. A similar problem of misdiagnosis is now taking place in the determination of Alzheimer's disease, which is often assigned as a convenient label without adequate evaluation. The types of depression seen by the Albany team did not fit well with the diagnostic categories in use. Therefore, it was not surprising that the professionals on the team did not always agree about diagnosis. However, there was usually consensus in identifying the social and health needs, and intervention planning in those areas became a cooperative experience. Geriatric clinicians continue to find that their diagnostic accuracy and effective treatment planning increase when open interchange about functional status and psychosocial correlates occurs, as staff communication may help to offset diagnostic uncertainty.

Results from the team were impressive. In a county of 35,000 persons over the age of 65, state hospital admissions in this cohort fell from an average of 25 per month to a total of 18 in a year. All of those admitted had major symptoms of mental illness; half of them were readmissions; and none had a primary problem of self-neglect. Of the remainder, many of whom were found to be self-neglecting, the majority stayed in their home environment and at discharge were felt to have improved in self-care (Vickers, 1976).

From their clinical experiences these staff established some knowledge about how to reverse patterns of self-neglect by attending to environmental changes and working to find supportive interventions that did not qualify as psychotherapy, but offered socialization supports and reduced isolation.

Gradually, in Albany County the practice of referring elderly patients for admission under the emergency mental health laws was replaced by consultation requests to the team. These began to be made by an ever widening variety of community resources. It appeared that despite the traditional pressures to admit, many workers in other agencies were more willing to request mental health consultation when they were reassured that commitment was not likely. The team was also asked to develop training for other community workers who wished to expand their knowledge of geropsychiatry, to improve their approach to older clients, and to enhance their ability to achieve satisfactory assessment outcomes without resorting to institutionalization or even requesting psychiatric consultation. This seemed to suggest that the team was now recognized as having more to offer than their powers of compulsory entry to a home or commitment to an institution (Woodruff et al., 1988).

Nonmobile psychogeriatric outpatient clinics with interdisciplinary staff can function like mobile teams, although they are limited by the willingness of clients to travel to them or the poor access to transportation, and they must still perform a home visit if the environmental conditions are to be adequately evaluated (Reifler and Eisdorfer, 1980).

CONCLUSION

At this time only a minority of community mental health centers comply with the most state-of-the-art approaches to psychogeriatrics. Up until the early 1980s, when community mental health centers were still under a mandate to offer specialized mental health services to aged persons, it looked as though major advances would be made in the quality and availability of mental health services to older people. This promised advance did not materialize, and today we see that problems of self-neglect are becoming further removed from the community mental health domain and being transferred to other delivery systems, such as adult protective service units under departments of social welfare.

If the current trend continues, community mental health agencies will have no significant role to play in geriatric mental health. Instead, geriatric mental health will be available through special diagnostic clinics that are being established in acute hospitals where the consequences of behavioral problems can be assigned some medical condition that warrants third-party payment for hospitalization. Those without insurance will continue to be without adequate mental and physical health care, and the risk and consequences of self-neglect will remain highest among those elderly with the fewest resources.

5

A Family Systems Perspective of Self-Neglect

Caroline T. Wilner and Nancy R. Vosler

Assessing self-neglect among the elderly from a family systems perspective increases the complexity of the issues but also provides a useful context for intervention that systematically broadens the store of available assessment information. The ethical analysis prepared by Cutler and Tisdale in this text, for example, incorporates a discussion of free will as it relates to the individual; however, the concept of free will can become problematic within the family because a systems framework describes a web of closely woven actions, reactions, and interactions that are both intra- and intergenerational. This chapter analyzes self-neglect in the context of family systems theory, family assessment, and intervention. A contextual framework that includes attention to life cycle stages provides a broader perspective for understanding self-neglect. Typologies of family behavior are applied to case study material. In the final section of the chapter, the authors provide generalized practice guidelines requiring further theoretical development and empirical study.

FAMILY SYSTEMS AND DEVELOPMENTAL PERSPECTIVES

Only recently have clinical gerontologists recognized the importance of drawing the family into the problem-solving efforts they undertake with or on behalf of elderly persons. Their family-directed interventions frequently apply a systems perspective and address transitional events that are part of the developmental cycles of the aging family. As background for considering the dynamics of self-neglect, this section summarizes the theories considered applicable to broad psychosocial behavioral concerns that may or may not impinge on the problem of elder self-neglect.

The family, for the purpose of this discussion, is a "grouping that consists of two or more individuals who define themselves as a family and who over time assume those obligations to one another that are generally considered an essential component of family systems" (NASW, 1982). Family units include biological family and extended family members by marriage(s) and common law relationships and even members of friendship networks that extend over time and come to be defined as "family." This expanded view of the family has important implications for work with self-neglecting elders who have never married, with no living children, and/or who have lost contact with family members and have become isolated.

Clinical application of a family systems perspective based on general systems (Bertalanffy, 1968) and social systems theory (Anderson and Carter, 1984) shifts the focus of diagnosis and treatment from the individual to the family and the wider social environment. A family is seen as a system of interacting persons, organized with boundaries and subsystems that often include marital and sibling subsystems as well as parent-offspring dyads. Patterns of communication and organization, including family rules and roles, emerge and change with time. The family system affects and is affected by members within the system and by the larger social systems in which it is embedded, for example, kinship and friendship networks, organizations and formal service delivery systems, and cultural and ethnic value systems within the community.

Implicit in the systemic view of the family is the idea of a "steady state," defined as a "total condition of the system in which it is in balance both internally and with its environment" (Anderson and Carter, 1984, p. 233). This steady state emerges with time such that family members know what to expect, how to act and react, and what is valued and forbidden. For the most part these understandings are basic and a somewhat constant part of daily life, but these can change. Some of the most universal and difficult transitions can best be understood in the context of the developmental life cycle stages of the family. Like individuals, families move through a series of developmental stages and tasks, from "unattached young adults" to "family in later life" (Carter and McGoldrick, 1988). Thus, families are social units created in a variety of expanding and contracting configurations that shift according to predictable and unpredictable crises and events. Families develop patterns of coping and resolution over the years, and these are applied in the aging process.

When does the final stage of the family life cycle begin and what are the developmental tasks of the aging family? Havighurst (1951) noted that the last developmental task of middle age is to adjust to aged parents so that both parent and middle-aged child adapt in a satisfactory manner. In this regard, most families in later life have a number of developmental transitions and tasks to negotiate, including launching of children, retirement, widowhood, grandparenthood, illness, dependency, and death. These experiences change the nature of parent-child relationships, and "the diversity, complexity, and importance of family relations in later life can be expected to become even greater in the future" (Walsh, 1988, p. 326).

The most difficult of the aging life cycle tasks involve illness, functional dependency, and death. Fears of losing cognitive and physical capacity are predominant themes among the elderly with consequences for intergenerational family relationships. These conditions test the hierarchical boundaries between aged parents and adult children. Williamson (1981) suggested that there has been no recognition of a crucial and transitional family task, which involves the termination of hierarchical boundaries between the first and second generations.

Clinicians may be overlooking the impact of the intergenerational confusion and ambivalence in the caregiver-carereceiver relationship during transitional periods. In the midst of confused roles, questions of power, autonomy, need, and parental omnipotence get raised and may produce intimidation and power struggles within the aging family. Power and the inability to renegotiate it may be one of the contributing factors in cases of self-neglect, as well as one of the variables in its prevention and elimination.

Williamson (1981) maintained that there should be radical renegotiation of power across generational boundaries. It is in this stage of the family life cycle that the uses and sources of relational power need to be reviewed and eventually redistributed in a more equalitarian direction. In the chaos of family dysfunction such redistribution may be impossible if members are struggling to maintain the old balance. These dynamics are clearly present in the family life of many self-neglecting elders. A vicious circle gets played out, as adult children struggle to hold on to the parent figure and, in the process, reject the "human" aspect of the parent that may desperately need help.

Prevailing patterns in U.S. families indicate that for the most part the elderly continue to be connected to their families in important ways. Adult children are not the only connection, as siblings and other relatives also provide a frequent flow of help and support. The dominant family for today may be, in fact, the modified extended family (Miller, 1981). It is the nature of the relationship through which the elderly are connected with society that determines whether they will be able to have a meaningful and secure life in the community.

What happens, however, to isolated older adults who have no kin and who are limited in their ability to utilize resources either through cognitive and physical impairments or through environmental factors that serve to reinforce the cause of their isolation? Rathbone-McCuan and Hashimi (1982) have suggested that isolation is a process in which the elderly lose their sense of personal integrity and link to social resources. As a result they may modify their expectations for successful living or respond by self-neglect, withdrawal, and possible drug or alcohol abuse.

In today's society, many elders can be physically and/or emotionally distant from biological family members. Some may be embedded in nontraditional families involving close friends or community resources. Such nontraditional family groupings are often created through necessity and are essential for the survival and well-being of that individual. Thus a group of friends in a retirement village, fellow members of a religious organization, or community caregivers, such as a visiting nurse, may function as a member of an extended family for an elder or an elderly couple who may be living alone. Homeless elderly can also form an informal survival network that serves as family. These nontraditional families extend friendship, caregiving, and support. When problems arise in these relationships as a result of changes in membership or through difficulties in communication, self-neglecting behaviors may signal a need for shifts in the system. It is perhaps this population, more than any other, that is at greatest risk for self-neglect.

In summary, family system and family life cycle perspectives shift the focus of problem description, assessment, and intervention from the individual elder to the family as a system, including the impact of larger social systems on the family unit. Although the majority of assessment and intervention models were originally developed from work with families with children, including adolescents, practitioners are beginning to apply the family life cycle perspective to families in later life with appropriate modifications in the phases of problem assessment and intervention planning.

Family Focused Assessment of Elder Self-Neglect

When confronting issues of self-neglect, the practitioner is faced with very critical and complex assessment and intervention decisions regarding elders and their families. As noted by Vickers in a previous chapter, multidisciplinary and interdisciplinary assessments are necessary in order to evaluate the physical, mental, and social well-being of the older adult. These approaches can also be of great benefit to the family. Measurement instruments are helpful in that they are "organizers, capable of turning amorphous and expansive goals into defined tasks and are a means by which progress or lack of progress is noted" (Kane and Kane, 1981).

The human element, however, is most important in the assessment of self-neglect because what is visible in a measure may screen out or act as a distraction from other important data, which can sometimes be read between the lines, and which can identify self-neglect as a risk or reality. The self-neglecting elder and his or her family are a puzzle where many different pieces must be fitted together to form a total picture. Assessment involves a combination of objective and subjective indicators, and in order to be genuine, evaluation should be not only scientific but also compassionate (Holman, 1983). A good evaluation should not only present hard facts but should also bring the patient to life from many different perspectives. This takes a discerning eye for detail, an ear for nuances, and a generous measure of intuition. It also involves self-awareness and insights into the practitioner's own personal dilemmas, ethical and religious learnings, judgmental values, and deep-rooted fears.

Assessment of the elderly individual must include a thorough and comprehensive evaluation of the elder's family. An understanding of how a family operates as a system is crucial because family systems are the basic social units to which most elders are connected to a greater or lesser degree. By adopting a systemic concept of the family, it is assumed that people do not operate as a collection of individuals but rather as part of a living and autonomous organism where rules, roles, structures, and processes exist that affect the individual member and the entire entity. The assessment process must not involve placing blame, per se, onto the elder or family. Rather than placing blame onto the older adult, the caregiver, or the resource agency, it becomes necessary to focus on those factors that sabotage adequate provision of elder services and impede the efforts of caregivers.

Components of the Assessment Process

Dubin (1987) developed a typology of conditions that contribute to the failure of caregiving systems associated with elder self-neglect. Four of the five categories, excluding the self-interested caregiver, are applicable to this discussion. These categories are the overwhelmed caregiving system, the elder refusing assistance, the dysfunctional caregiving system, and the elder alone. Three cases have been selected to reflect all of these categories except the elder who refuses assistance, but such an individual is described elsewhere in the text.

To complete an assessment that is more or less applicable to each of these categories, the family environment encompassing physical/financial resources and social-emotional support, intergenerational history focusing on themes and relationship issues, family organizational structure, and communication patterns must be included (Hartman and Laird, 1983; Kolevzon and Green, 1985). Each of these components will be summarized.

Family Environment

System theory focuses on the impact of available resources, resource deficits, crises, and external events in the wider social environment for family functioning. Within the ecological environment (Hartman and Laird, 1983), two aspects that are often of critical importance are physical and financial resources and social-emotional support. Interventions within the environment may in some cases be all that are needed to change self-neglect behaviors and enable the reestablishment of functional potential for individuals and family.

For any family system to function as effectively as possible, adequate resources must be available to meet members' basic survival needs. Assessment of self-neglect behavior needs to include exploration of possible resource deficits for the elder within the context of his or her current family. For many families, self-neglect signals that family network survival needs are overwhelming current residential and financial resources. System theory posits that change in one part of the system will create changes in other parts of the system; thus, if housing and/or financial stress is contributing to self-neglect, these needs must be addressed immediately. If there is no direct linkage of these resource deficits to elder self-neglect, efforts to meet basic needs are still of primary concern.

Social-emotional support, or its lack, available to the family and particularly to the primary caregiver(s) is a focal aspect of assessment. In self-neglect situations there may be a lack of reciprocity. This may manifest in such situations as a lack of expressed gratitude directed to the caregiver, misperceptions of the caregiver's motivation, a reductionistic attitude about the elder's capabilities, or a failure to seek the elder's approval for caregiving activities. Social and emotional exchanges that do not enhance personal need, sometimes unspoken or unrecognized, may feed into and escalate the self-neglect drama.

Intergenerational History

Family intergenerational history, including themes and relationships issues, should be covered in an assessment to determine their relevance for intervention. Bowen (1978; see also Kerr and Bowen, 1988) developed an approach to work with families that is applicable to our perspective on self-neglect. There may be patterned interaction such as those developed to cope with chronic stress or enmeshment within consecutive generations that produce rigid behavior prescriptions such as self-neglect. Poulshock and Deimling (1984) suggested that caregiver burden is an individualized response to specific caregiving contexts.

Among self-neglecting elders and their families, the greatest subjective burden may involve feelings of helplessness and rage. These may be intensified by role conflict, financial and physical burdens, fatigue, and feelings of guilt and inadequacy. Related interventions may include lowering emotional reactivity, strengthening problem-solving ability, enhancing differentiation of self, and modifiying relationships within the extended system, including repairing cut-offs (Walsh, 1982). These strategies are applied to self-neglect both as a serious and immediate problem and as indicative of a relationship(s) dysfunction. Some of these techniques may also have lasting positive consequences for multiple generations in the family system.

Family Structure

The structural/strategic model of family therapy, based on the work of Haley and Minuchin, focuses more explicitly and exclusively on current family functioning (Kolevzon and Green, 1985). This model assumes that healthy families have clear and firm boundaries, that they are organized in generational hierarchies, that coalitions across generational boundaries are dysfunctional and can result in systems that communicate dysfunction, that healthy functioning involving flexibility within the system enables individual growth and change, that incorporation of both autonomy and interdependence are critical, and that both system continuity and adaptive restructuring in response to changing developmental and environmental demands are important and possible (Walsh, 1982). Intervention may, for example, facilitate family role negotiation so that an impaired elder shifts from an inappropriate child position to egalitarian mutual elder-caregiver problem solving.

Family Communications

In the communication model developed by Satir (1988), systems are viewed as "nonverbal messages in reaction to current communication dysfunction" (Walsh, 1982, p. 27). Positive family functioning entails establishing an open system in which self-esteem of members is high, communication is direct, clear, and cogent, and family rules are explicit, appropriate, and can be changed when the need arises (Satir, 1988). In contrast, low self-esteem families often develop rigid interaction patterns with unclear, unspecific, and incongruent communication; their rules often are covert, fixed, inhumane, and dated. In such families a symptom such as self-neglecting behavior may be a nonverbal "cry for help" on behalf of both the individual and the family system.

Characteristics of the intervention derived from this model include maximum involvement of numbers of family members, emphasis on the development of clear communication, and sharing family experiences. The practitioner's primary assessment tool is identification of confusing and incongruent verbal and nonverbal messages, identification of feelings of low self-worth, and verification of implicit and/or unconscious family roles, rules, secrets, and interaction patterns. The assessment process is also an opportunity for a practitioner's participation with the family in a change process where the role includes modeling communication, enabling appropriate family roles and rule formulation, and facilitating connection with the family to enhance individual positive growth and self-esteem.

Family Assessment Tools

A number of assessment tools have been developed in conjunction with several of these modes of family intervention. Hartman and Laird (1983) developed the eco-map as a tool to objectify resources available to and being used by the family, resources that are in short supply or not available, and the types of interactions that occur between resource systems and family members or the family as a whole. For example, the relationship between the family and specific social welfare agencies and organizations can be discussed and mapped to answer questions about benefits and service abilities of the extended family and formal network to provide assistance to help resolve crisis. The strengths of these connections for problem solving can also be examined.

An assessment tool used extensively with the intergenerational model of family practice is the genogram (Bowen, 1978; Hartman and Laird, 1983), which identifies multiple generations in the family tree and tracks their events, losses, emotional cut-offs, and relationship patterns and issues. This assessment device can engage the elderly client in the beginning of a life review process, identify significant family members with whom connections might be able to be reestablished, and track emotional and relationship issues that might have some bearing on the self-neglecting behavior.

Another tool used particularly with the structural model of family-centered practice is family mapping. After identifying the current members and engaging as many of them as possible in the assessment interview, the practitioner observes, maps, and tests alliances, coalitions, power hierarchies, unclear or rigid boundaries, triangles, conflict relationships, and executive and other subsystems (Minuchin, 1974). Hypotheses concerning family functioning are developed, and strategies for family system reorganization are planned (Haley, 1987). Although the symptom is taken seriously as a communication of family dysfunction, the focus of intervention is the family system itself, based on the practitioner's knowledge of organization and structure.

Case Illustrations

The following typical cases were selected to show the multiple patterns of self-neglect within the family system. Each applies some of the information provided on assessment of the dynamics within and across generations. The first case illustrates the isolated elder and applies an eco-map (Figure 5.1) for displaying the role of the informal system that surrounds the isolated elder. The second case illustrates a dysfunctional family (Figure 5.2) where relationship conflicts cutting across generations illuminate the context of self-neglecting behaviors. The third case displays a much broader caregiving system that includes both the family and the community network. (Figure 5.3).

Isolated Elder

Paul and Irene V are an elderly couple who have been married for over 50 years and who live together in a two-family home in a city in Ohio. Paul, age 84, and Irene, age 81, live in the upstairs flat, and tenants rent the downstairs apartment. They have never had children, and

FIGURE 5.1
The Isolated Elder

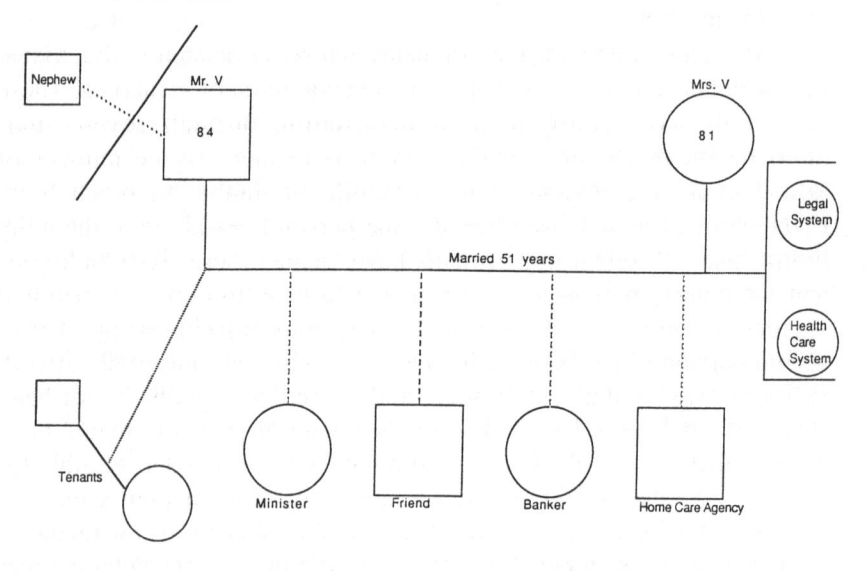

their only living relative is a nephew who lives over 80 miles away. Both were active and successful business people who continued to work until they were in their 70s. After retirement they were involved with church, clubs, and organizational work. Mrs. V became demented about four years ago, but it was a gradual onset, and Mr. V was able to manage his wife relatively well. It wasn't until three years later that the impairment became noticeably worse. But by the time church members and neighbors became aware of the couple's deficits, both of them were severely demented. A concerned church friend, who had known the couple for nearly 50 years, initiated a referral for assessment of the situation.

The couple had no services coming into the house, and Mr. V was attempting to manage the house and to care for his wife by himself. He still drove to the supermarket twice a week but was frequently getting lost. The tenant downstairs had to look for him on several occasions. Spoiled food was found in the trunk of the car, food that Mr. V had forgotten was there. Mrs. V, tiny and emaciated, barely ate and could not express hunger. She apparently had been subsisting on a diet of yogurt, bananas, and rolls, the primary foods that her husband brought home, and she still smoked cigarettes, which he purchased for her. Burn marks on the carpets and furniture were evident throughout the house.

Mrs. V was unable to do anything and spent most of her time packing all her clothing and belongings into boxes, which her husband then unpacked at the end of the day. The house was littered with packed cartons and trails of soiled clothing. At first Mr. V helped his wife with bathing, but clearly she had not bathed in many weeks. She has been incontinent of both stool and urine, and the house reeked of excrement. Mr. V had been leaving his wife when he went out, and although she had difficulty managing stairs, she had on occasions gotten out and wandered. The tenants had found Mrs. V walking about nude or semidressed, at times hallucinating and confused.

Mr. V has become extremely paranoid and accused friends of breaking into the apartment and taking things. As a result, he was often up all night "keeping guard" against intruders. He had not slept in his bed in weeks but slept in snatches in an armchair and kept a billy club on hand. He had expressed a desire to die and had threatened to drive into a nearby lake. He had also started drinking at night to calm his nerves, and the tenants had found empty liquor bottles in the stairwell.

The only person with any influence was their banker, who had had power of attorney for several months. This had been initiated by the nephew to help the couple pay their bills. The banker prepared the checks which Mr. V signed, but it was a haphazard system because Mr. V was unable to keep track of bills and many had gone unpaid.

The Dysfunctional Family

Mr. W is an 81-year-old married male who lives alone in a small apartment in an East Coast city. He has been living alone for a year and a half, ever since his wife of 56 years was admitted to a nursing home because of severe impairment from Alzheimer's disease. He has a long history of multiple medical problems, which have been progressive. These include congestive heart failure, hypertension, diabetes, dizziness, chest pains, and hearing loss. He also has a history of depression with suicidal intentions. He has on numerous occasions expressed a wish to die, saying that his life is miserable and that he wishes that it could be over.

Mr. W is a former salesman who retired at the age of 62 because of ill health and his inability to stand on his feet for any length of time. Work was his only outlet for socialization, and after retirement he became increasingly reclusive and unwilling to leave his apartment. Before his wife became ill, she managed some of his care needs, although her skills in managing were marginal, and both lived in a precarious environment. Mr. W continued to resist recommended therapies, would not follow his

82 / SELF-NEGLECTING ELDERS

FIGURE 5.2
The Dysfunctional Family

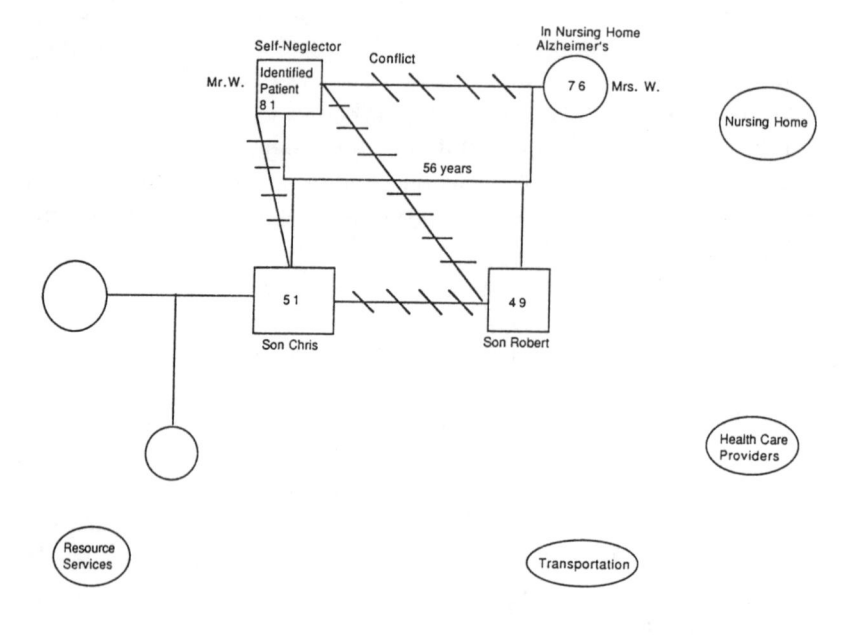

prescribed diet, and would rarely leave the house. Their marital relationship had always been strained with a long history of hostility and anger yet followed a pattern of manipulation and dependence.

The family consisted of two sons, Chris, age 51, and Robert, age 49. Chris was married and had one daughter. Robert had never married. Both sons remember constant fighting between the parents, with suicide as a constant manipulative threat by the father. They had been terrorized for years by his violent behavior and his lengthy "black" moods, which would last for many weeks. As a result, they had distanced themselves from both parents for many years and only became involved again after their mother began showing cognitive impairment and was diagnosed with Alzheimer's disease. The relationship between the siblings had also been historically poor, full of resentments and unresolved rivalries.

Mr. W's self-neglecting behavior rapidly became life threatening following his wife's placement. He had had several falls that resulted in injuries, including scalp lacerations and multiple bruises. His legs had become swollen, and at home he wore no shoes most of the time. He was unable to get in and out of a bathtub, and his personal hygiene habits had deteriorated to an indifferent sponge bath once in a while, and he had stopped shaving. His clothing was soiled, and his general appearance was unkempt and dirty. Medication compliance was questionable at best. Mr. W's diet was poor, although his appetite improved dramatically when one of the sons brought food or was able to persuade him to go out for a meal.

Although his children were alarmed and concerned by their father's self-neglecting situation, they felt immobilized by their feelings of distaste for his bitterness, rage, and frequent complaints about how terrible things were, particularly because he refused to accept any changes and would not tolerate their well-meaning suggestions. They continued to turn on each other with blame and recriminations, as they became increasingly frustrated by their feelings of helplessness and growing stress.

Overwhelmed Caregiving System

Mrs. M, an obese 82-year-old widow, with multiple problems of diabetes, hypertension, incontinence, and frequent falls, lives alone in a Northeastern city, in a one-bedroom subsidized senior citizens' apartment building where she moved five years after her husband's death. It seemed to be an appropriate move and an ideal solution for an elderly woman left

FIGURE 5.3
Overwhelmed Caregiving System

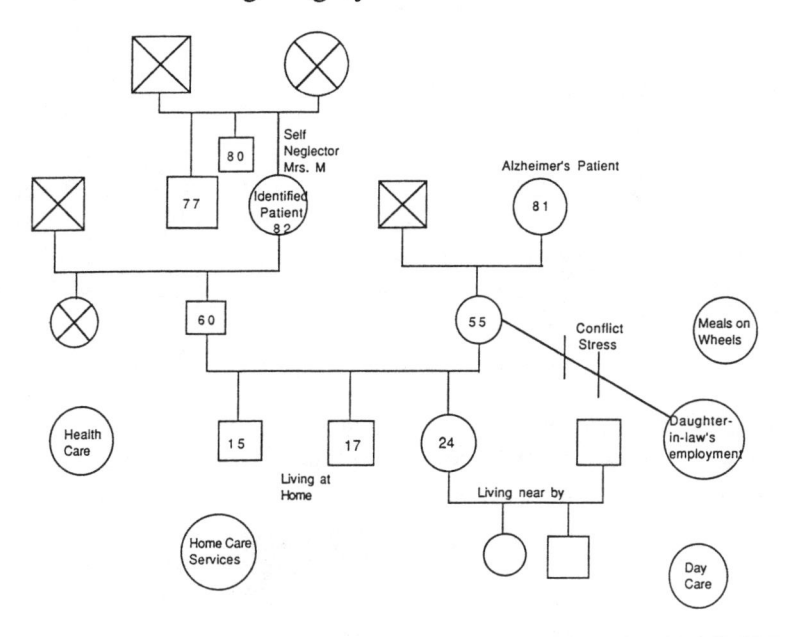

alone, who was alert and sought to maintain her independence. Yet the ideal solution culminated in a disastrous reality as Mrs. M refused to avail herself of the available supportive services in the building, such as meals and socialization, and began a downward course of self-neglect.

Her family consisted of a son, age 60, a daughter-in-law who worked full time, and two elderly brothers, age 80 and 77, who had severe health problems of their own. In the course of the past four years, she had adamantly and consistently refused all help from outside agencies in terms of personal or chore services, had refused to eat in the dining room or to have meals delivered, and had only reluctantly gone to a doctor for health maintenance and follow-up for her diabetes. Her falls had increased dramatically over the period of a year, and twice she had been unable to get up and lay all night on the floor before she was found the next day by her daughter-in-law.

Her appearance was unkempt, and she had extremely edematous legs. Her personal hygiene had deteriorated, and because she was unable to get in and out of the bathtub independently, she had not bathed in many months other than a sketchy sponge bath. Her son and daughter-in-law had complained about the disorder in her apartment, but "disorder" was a gross minimization of the chaos that was evident. Nearly every inch of space was littered with old newspapers, clothing, boxes of possessions, knick-knacks, old letters, and what appeared to be trash. The bed was piled high with clothes and papers, and it was evident that Mrs. M had not slept in her bed for many months. Instead, she had made a nest for herself on the corner of the couch and dozed at odd hours so that her days and nights were often confused. The apartment smelled from episodes of incontinence, and roaches rustled in the stacks of yellowed newspapers. Her kitchen was empty of all foods except for a bag of sweet potatoes, a jar of peanut butter, a half loaf of bread, a bottle of soured milk, and a large container of prepared cake icing, which she liked to eat with a spoon. The refrigerator also contained four bottles of insulin and some syringes. Three of the bottles were outdated, and it did not appear that the fourth bottle had ever been used.

Discussion of Cases

Although the case of Mrs. M is one of the most dramatic and obvious examples, self-neglect comes in many packages and varieties. It is often a hazy and ambiguous area, implying free will, yet clearly collusive in that family and institutions are generally helpless in preventing or intervening in the self-neglecting and destructive patterns of behavior, yet they often contribute directly or indirectly to that behavior as did Mr. W's sons who argued endlessly over responsibility for his care. It is a particularly frustrating and confusing area of elder care, subject to ambiguous definitions and confusing assessments.

From a family systems perspective, we cannot isolate the focus of self-neglect on the self-neglectful individual alone. Paradoxically we must also focus on other neglecters as well. By doing so, however, we further blur the boundaries between the concept of neglect and self-neglect and begin to flounder in the complex issues of self-determination, free will, benign or malevolent intent, and free judgment. In the process of identifying and assessing the self-neglecting elderly, we must also identify who and what neglecters are operative. What part does the neglecter play in the complex pattern of self-neglect? And how do we as health professionals and those in protective services differentiate between the fine lines of neglect in order to initiate constructive interventions?

The definition of self-neglect is ambiguous and paradoxical in that it implies free will. Yet from a family systems perspective, the concept of free will is in itself ambiguous because systems thinking indicates and describes a web of closely woven actions, reactions, and interactions that are both intra- and intergenerational. The case of Mr. and Mrs. V clearly demonstrates these complexities when the numerous, but uncoordinated, efforts of an out-of-town nephew, a banker, the health-care and legal systems, and a tenant are all failing to resolve the neglectful situation.

Although Mrs. M's situation was clearly a case of self-neglect that was quickly spiraling toward a life-threatening crisis, it was equally clear that in her case, as in most cases, a family drama was being played out, a drama in which each family member played an important role in contributing toward the self-neglecting behavior. Although the key and strongest player was Mrs. M herself, the list of neglecters included her son and daughter-in-law, her brothers, her physician, the manager of the senior citizens building where she lived, and, in some fashion, each failed agency with which she had had contact over the recent years. Overtly and covertly, each joined in some fashion in aiding and abetting the self-destructive pattern of behavior.

Perhaps the greatest obstacle toward effective intervention is the issue of opposing perceptions. As Parsons and Cox (1989) have pointed out, decision making then becomes unharmonious necessitating empowerment and family mediation. Empirical evidence now exists to indicate that generational differences in perception are a common problem in caregiving efforts. Townsend and Poulshock (1986) discuss some of the theoretical arguments that help explain the differences. They point out the unique role of the elder for whom the helping network is egocentrically focused.

Thus, Mr. W becomes the focal point of change efforts that in actuality involve three additional family members. Several health-care providers focus on Mr. W and relief of the self-neglect while the other family issues continue to confound these efforts at intervention. It is the elder who theoretically has the first-hand knowledge of need; the adult child occupies both an insider and outsider role. Salend's (1984, p. 66) statement of "one man's self-neglect may be another's exercise of free judgement" is an accurate and frustrating conflict of professional duty and judgment in which choices often have to be made between the need to intervene in self-destructive behavior and the patient's right to self-determination.

The drama of this conflict is most poignantly played out within the family arena, where moral principles and divided loyalties are governed by the culture, rules, language, and history of each family. Many factors influence the exercise of autonomy. Perceptions of need are often intricately interwoven with perceptions of power and autonomy. A consideration of the values at play as well as the diverse cultural and educational backgrounds is crucial in understanding discrepant perceptions.

Mrs. M came from a background where female dominance and strength were key family components. A daughter is now dead, but both daughter and son had respected Mrs. M's power and almost never went against her expressed wishes. Her surviving son continued to see her in the role that she had played all her life and that his grandmother and great-aunts had played before her. Within her own nuclear family, his wife was also the dominant figure, and he found himself caught between two powerful women who were often in conflict with each other. Mrs. M's daughter-in-law felt that the only solution was a nursing home placement and was angry that her husband was unwilling to initiate such a placement. She had broached the subject with her mother-in-law on several occasions and had met with hostility and extreme resistance.

Mrs. M's primary perception of need was to be left alone in order to live her life without interference. That need took precedence over all others and distorted her perception of her present lifestyle. Where others saw chaos, she saw her own personal order. Mrs. M's daughter-in-law viewed the patient's needs quite differently. By providing minimal help only, the daughter-in-law contributed to the self-neglecting behavior, thus convincing herself even further that the best place for Mrs. M was a nursing home where others could supervise her care. Rather than fight with her mother-in-law or make an effort to understand, it was easier to comply with the patient's wishes, for example, providing her with inappropriate foods when she shopped for her.

The problems confronting agencies and practitioners are equally confusing when it comes to self-neglecting behaviors. Although mandatory reporting laws exist in most states, older adults are considered responsible for themselves unless declared incompetent in court. Physicians, nurses, social workers, housing managers, home health aides, and other health professionals or even volunteers can easily perceive the dangers of self-neglecting behaviors, but their subsequent stance is generally frustration, anger, and a punitive attitude of "either do as I say, or we will take away your rights." Cajoling, threats, and angry behavior serve to accent the conflict so that a power struggle quickly becomes evident.

In truth, formal services often are unsuccessful and rejected by both the patient and the caregivers, particularly if the formal service is introduced as a panacea for the stressful situation and put into the home without an appropriate and skilled evaluation to determine how it can be incorporated to the best functioning of both. Frequently, no effort is made to ascertain why a patient or family does or does not accept formal services, yet such information can be critical in utilizing the most effective strategies to help impaired and frail elderly. One sample study of caregiver supports pointed out that acceptance of formal supports may not necessarily mean that the person is content with the situation but rather accepts it only because no other alternatives are apparent (Hawranik, 1985). If the entire caregiving situation is not then carefully explored, failure becomes inevitable.

CONCLUSION

This chapter has attempted to demonstrate the basic premise that work with the elderly cannot be separated from work with the family and ecological system. The application of this thesis is perhaps most powerfully seen in the areas of elder self-neglect, where every resource becomes a critical factor in the survival of the individual. Often the resource is not lacking, but the fundamental effectiveness of the system is jeopardized by dysfunctional patterns and lack of organizational cohesion. The incorporation of the family systems perspective into assessment and treatment planning will assist the practitioner in identifying strengths and weaknesses and gaining a more comprehensive perspective of the self-neglecting elderly person.

Unfortunately much of current practice with the elderly focuses almost exclusively on the individual. Family therapy literature itself is only now beginning to look at and theorize the later stages of the family life cycle and how it impacts on family dynamics and dysfunctional behaviors. We know now that the stereotypical notion that most elderly are isolated from their families is simply not true. Most elders also appear to have a network of support intact even if biologic ties are lacking. It is critical for practitioners to be aware of and explore these nonbiologic kinships in order to effectively utilize strategies to help the self-neglecting person. It is necessary to see all players as part of a system, otherwise strategies become jeopardized as the system becomes unbalanced in the change process.

Furthermore, the interplay between the health-care system and the family system of which the elder is a member will continue to be critical as the rising tide of elder population within ever shrinking resources may put an increasing number of elderly at risk for self-neglect. The family is and will continue to be the most important resource for its elders. It has been so throughout history. Self-neglect is not just "self-neglect" but part of a larger picture that includes multiple family actors. Although the issues that may lead to elder self-neglect remain the same, a changing perspective may facilitate better approaches to meeting those issues.

III

SPECIAL RISKS AND SUBGROUPS

6

Institutional Care Settings and Self-Neglect

Joan K. Hashimi and Linda Withers

Self-neglect in an institution is not a readily understood concept. The nursing home, mental hospital, and boarding home are seen as answers to the problem of self-neglect in the community. The common perception is that any elder care needs not being met in the community will be provided in an institution, thus relieving the elder from responsibility for personal care. Yet, in institutions, maintaining or improving self-care skills is central to maximizing the elders' autonomy and control; both vital keys to life satisfaction.

With advancing age there is increasing probability that an individual will be confronted with an ever more complex self-care regime and fewer resources to meet care needs. For some elders, a time comes when care needs overwhelm their personal resources; when that happens assistance becomes necessary. For most elders, a personal resource deficit is compensated for by family and, in many cases, supplemented by other community-based caregivers. If the amount of added help required by the elder is too great and family care providers cannot meet the need or if no family care provider exists or is available and community-based care is unavailable, institutional care is necessary to maintain the elder's optimal health and well-being. There is a range of institutional settings: group homes, boarding homes, mental hospitals, and nursing homes (intermediate care facilities and skilled nursing facilities). Depending on the elder's mental and physical functional capacity, he or she can be best matched to one of these facilities. In this chapter, we focus on the nursing home. The authors explore self-neglect in the nursing home and measures the staff can adopt to minimize its occurrence.

THE NURSING HOME

The nursing home itself is an institution in crisis. Nursing homes today are facing increased numbers needing placement, increased costs of care, decreased Medicaid funds, increasing levels of debility of incoming residents, and increasing scrutiny by legislators, families, and citizen groups to assure that quality care is provided (Shaughnessy, 1989). Nursing homes meet these demands with direct services staff that have minimal training. Staffing needs are complicated by a high rate of staff burnout and turnover (Burda, 1987; Reagan, 1986).

We presently have 19,100 nursing homes with a total of 1,624,200 beds, representing a 22-percent increase in homes and a 38-percent increase in beds from 1974. Of these homes, 75 percent are for-profit; 20 percent, nonprofit; and 5 percent are governmentally operated (Strahan, 1987). In 1985, Medicaid paid for about 42 percent of nursing home costs, $14.7 billion, which is about one-third of all Medicaid expenditures (Burda, 1987). In contrast, Medicare paid for approximately 2 percent of the nation's nursing home expenditures (U.S. GAO, 1986). The large percentage of nursing home costs paid by governmental funds makes any reduction of those funds, as is now being suggested, quite significant in nursing home management (Burda, 1987).

Combined with threats to financial supports is the gradual decline in the condition of clients at their points of entry into the home. The new residents are increasingly more debilitated. One can presume their medical care needs will be increasingly more complex (Hing, 1987).

In addition, the numbers of people needing nursing home placement will more than likely increase in the coming years because the over-85 cohort is the fastest growing segment of the population. The over-85 cohort will triple between 1980 and 2010, from 2.2 million to 6.1 million (U.S. Senate Special Committee on Aging, 1989). Although at any given time, only 5 percent of all people over 65 years of age are in a nursing home, the lifetime chances for nursing home placement for anyone over 65 is a topic of considerable debate (Liang and Jow-Ching Fu, 1986; McConnel, 1984; Palmore, 1976). The estimates of the lifetime risk of a nursing home stay range from 25 percent to 50 percent. A document released by the Select Committee on Aging (1985) states that the prevalence rates for nursing home use are 0.5 percent for those 65–74, 5 percent to 6 percent for those 75–84, and approximately 22 percent for those 85 and older. They also state that the lifetime risk for nursing home placement is 25 percent.

The typical nursing home resident is over 80 years of age, white (73 percent), a woman (about 75 percent), and widowed, divorced, or never married (86 percent). Many have no surviving children or children who are working and/or live in other areas of the country. It has been estimated that 60 percent to 80 percent have some form of cognitive impairment that limits functional and/or social abilities. In addition 75 percent are estimated to have mental disorders or behavioral problems that include depressed withdrawn behavior, agitation, nervousness, or abusive and disruptive behavior. Tranquilizers are given to 49 percent of residents, and 34.4 percent are given hypnotic sedatives (Hing, 1981; Hing, 1987). Use of these medications has come under increased scrutiny; their use may be unwarranted and may interfere with self-care (Canti and Korek, 1987; Smith, 1990).

The number of nursing home residents who are self-neglectful has not been documented, but we do have some data on self-injury, which appears an overlapping concept. Mishara and Kastenbaum (1973) reported that in a nursing home setting they observed 70 percent of those on a female ward and 44 percent on a male ward engaged in self-injurious behaviors. The lower percentage on male wards can be explained by the fact that on the male wards approximately half were restrained to prevent self-injury. Of those not restrained 76 percent engaged in self-injurious acts. Rovner et al. (1986) noted that 14 percent of their subjects engaged in self-destructive behavior. However, they also noted that 38 percent were passive-aggressive. Favazza (1989), in a study of self-mutilation, reports incidence numbers for the general population of mentally retarded groups at 0.75 percent and 13.6 percent. It may be that if agreement were reached on what acts were self-neglectful or self-injurious, these estimates would be closer. There does seem to be evidence that this is a serious problem for institutionalized elders.

DEFINING SELF-NEGLECT

Defining self-neglect within the nursing home requires something beyond the definition suitable to the community; that is, a failure to provide for oneself appropriate nutrition, clothing, housing, social activities, or medical/psychological services. Within the nursing home, all of these basic needs must be provided by legal mandate. Indeed, persons who are deemed unable or unwilling to conform to acceptable levels of self-care in community situations are placed in the nursing home for precisely that reason. There is an implicit assumption that, if you cannot or will not take care of yourself, you go into a nursing home, and the staff then care for you. This logic, therefore, suggests there can be no self-neglect because the resident is seldom held accountable. This logic holds only when considering health care as an undivided unit, that is, if one were to perceive self-care as a whole that one could provide totally for oneself or not be able to provide for oneself at all.

However, an individual within a nursing home may be able to fulfill some self-care needs and may be expected to do so. Thus, one could modify the above definition of neglect by adding "the failure of the elder to assume responsibility for those aspects of self-care that he or she is still able to provide." Examples of self-neglect would include

  refusing treatment, for example, refuse to eat adequately, refuse medications;
  neglecting proper precautions, for example, wear nonskid slippers rather than just socks; and
  actively harming self, for example, save up medications to take all at once, scratch at self, pull out tubes.

Self-neglect may not always be so easy to recognize or quite this obvious. Caregivers must begin to recognize more subtle signs. The following behaviors call for observations over time by individuals (staff and family) who are familiar with the elder and are sensitive to behavioral and physical change:

  weight loss or gain,
  reduced social activities,
  unreported bruises or scratches,
  demoralization, a giving up, and
  not reporting to staff health changes that may signal need for more extensive care.

These events are not always caused by self-neglect; they may result from undiscovered health problems. Each behavior should be carefully explored for its meaning for health care. Accurate assessment of each resident's behavior is prerequisite to designing an appropriate response. This assessment is a challenge to the skills and experience of nursing home staff.

An issue that arises in defining self-neglect is whether it is intentional. If self-neglect is intentional, what motivates this behavior? More specifically, one must ask if the elder intended to do what he or she did knowing that the result would be self-harm. If the answer is yes, then could one imply suicidal intent? Kastenbaum and Mishara (1971) state that suicide is simply the most identifiable form of avoidable death in old age. They also speak of "subintentional suicide" and "life-threatening behavior" and suggest that deaths resulting from these behaviors equal or exceed the numbers of those who do commit suicide. They report evidence that those individuals who manifest a will to die, do indeed appear to die sooner than expected. In fact, little is known about suicidal intent in the elderly (Blazer, Bachar, and Manton, 1986).

Essentially, we are dealing with a question of whether an elder values his or her life in spite of impairment. In considering the degree to which life is valued, one must examine the differences in values, ethics, and beliefs that distinguish us all. The individuals who adjust well to life within the nursing home, for their own reasons, accept their limitations in functioning and find ways to continue for themselves a meaningful existence. In making this assertion, we are assuming that the nursing home is at least benign, if not an institution that supports meaningful social experience. For as Mishara, Robertson, and Kastenbaum (1973) have shown, self-injurious behavior is highly related to environmental factors. These environmental factors include the extent to which activities and social stimulation, opportunities for resident choice, and a staff sensitive to the needs of the patients are available (Folmer and Wilson, 1989; Mishara and Kastenbaum, 1973). For elders who do not value a continuation of life with drastic limitations in personal autonomy, self-destruction, or at least a disregard of behavioral consequences, is to be expected (Braun, Wykle, and Cowling, 1988). Additionally, unless a nursing home resident has been declared incompetent, he or she still has the right to refuse medical/psychological/social treatment. "Medical caregivers ... are not empowered under our laws to make formal determinations of 'competency,' nor can they automatically delimit individual rights based on medical assessments" (Zuckerman, 1987, p. 60).

Thus, providers are confronted with a Catch 22. If they force a resident beyond his or her will to do things that ensure survival, they violate the resident's rights of choice and add to the helplessness and loss of autonomy the client is experiencing. But, if the nursing home providers do not insist, they may well be legally liable because it is their mission to provide life-enhancing care.

A significant amount of research has been given to the phenomenon of translocation shock. Relocation from totally independent living to a more protective environment is disruptive to the elder and presses him or her to face the reality of physical and/or mental decline. Relocation represents an interrelated set of stressors that include the physical and/or mental decline and loss of a familiar environment and stabilizing routine. To these losses are added the demands of adjustment to the new environment (Butler and Lewis, 1982; Kasl et al., 1980). Studies reveal that a high percentage of individuals die within one year following placement in a nursing home or evidence higher rates of maladaptation (Lieberman and Tobin, 1983). For some new residents, who were moved to a nursing home in the terminal stages of an illness, this outcome should not be overinterpreted, but for others it may represent a response to involuntary relocation. If elders are institutionalized against their will, one can well expect responses not at all unlike those of other victims of severe psychological trauma, for example, hyperreactivity, explosive aggressive outbursts, acts of aggression against self or others, emotional constriction, and social isolation (Van der Kolk, 1987).

In some cases, neglect may be intentional but for reasons other than self-harm. There may be a conscious choice to be self-neglecting because of secondary gains. Institutionalization leaves little room for individuality. One finds various ways to retain self-worth and to have needs met. Self-neglecting behavior can result in increased attention. For example, refusal to eat results in increased assessment and intervention from nurses, physicians, dietitians, and ancillary staff. It can result in obtaining specially prepared food, including all one's favorites. Refusal to interact socially with other residents can result in frequent one-to-one visits by staff.

Self-neglect may be related to poor staff understanding of resident needs or careless, demeaning, inadequate, authoritarian, and/or mechanical provision of direct care services. In this instance, refusal to cooperate in self-care may be the resident's only way to fight back. Although this behavior may be self-injurious, it may be the resident's only way to gain some level of control or to seek attention. In some sense, this might be a sign of health. The resident has not given up a sense of self and a right of entitlement to appropriate care.

Rothbaum et al. (1982) suggest that the literature has become too focused on control being understood as active mastery over the environment. They define this as primary control; secondary control is a process in which the individual, after repeatedly failing, persists in certain inward behaviors that serve to provide perceived control. Illustrations of secondary control would include avoiding tasks at which they might fail to prevent disappointment or aligning with powerful others (for example, group involvement or religion). A religious response suggests events are in "God's hands." Indeed, there is a sense of mastery or control of self when one is able to accept adverse events interpreted as being out of one's hands. One must also remember that the elder may exercise the opportunity of being in control by choosing not to be in control (Rodin, 1986).

Lazarus and Folkman interpret dependent behaviors differently. They state, "It seems best to assume that aging per se brings no changes in coping; it is when people are faced with deteriorating environmental conditions and impaired physical and mental resources that they display regression to the more dependent, helpless period of infancy and early childhood" (1984, p. 173).

In some cases, personal values and beliefs may cause self-neglect to be defined differently. Religious beliefs may lead to fasting during holy periods. A solitary person may value time alone more than any social involvement. Indeed, if they had grown to enjoy solitude before entering the nursing home, having to share a room may be difficult enough without having to be socially involved during free time.

In trying to interpret self-neglecting behaviors, one should take care. One may be forcing overly complex interpretations on a human failing. We may all be guilty of sinking into dependency when someone is willing to provide a service that is troublesome to provide for ourselves (Booth, 1986).

In most cases, self-care will be complicated by cognitive impairment as a result of organic mental disorder. The definition of dementia (affecting in some degree up to two-thirds of all nursing home patients) states, "Impaired judgment and impulse control are common ... a previously neat and meticulous person [may] become slovenly and unconcerned about appearance. People with dementia may wander and become lost. They may occasionally do harm to themselves and others" (DSM-III R, 1987).

Defining self-neglect within an institution, it seems, is an exercise in separating those tasks of personal care that nursing home staff must carry out — because the resident is unable (as a result of organic and/or functional mental disorders or physical disability) to take responsibility for — from the items of self-care that the resident can accomplish. Thus, we would exclude from our definition of self-neglect harmful acts, omissions of self-care that could more clearly be described as suicidal, and responsibility for self-care tasks that the resident is not capable of performing or is learning to perform because of organic mental disorders or physical disease. To call behaviors self-neglecting when the person is unable to provide self-care, even with assistance and instruction, resembles blaming the victim.

SELF-NEGLECT IN THE NURSING HOME

Once one is institutionalized, the primary responsibility for care is shifted from the individual to the staff of the facility. A complete array of services designed to either promote or maintain the individual's physical and emotional health status is provided. Nursing homes can be viewed as being on a continuum of approaches to resident care, from the protective to the supportive. In the protective model, employees do what is seen as best for the resident. In the supportive model, the emphasis is on enabling the resident to provide as much self-care as possible (Booth, 1986).

Within both models, the resident still retains some control. Table 6.1 depicts services provided by the nursing home and behaviors the individual may exhibit that can complicate the care. The following case example illustrates these possibilities.

Mr. Smith is 74 years old and has resided in a nursing home for about 2-1/2 years. He was admitted to the nursing home following a hospitalization for an above-the-knee amputation. His wife had died approximately two years earlier, very unexpectedly. As stated in the social history, "He had been very neglectful of himself since her death. It was difficult to ascertain whether his neglect was due to lack of know-how or apathy or both." Mr. Smith, a severe diabetic, ignored his diet and health in general. Before the recent amputation, he underwent a partial left foot amputation. His home was filthy, and his personal hygiene practices were poor at best. He ate primarily snack food, which did not comply with his diabetic diet.

His father and several brothers also had severe diabetes, and all had amputations. He has been fearful most of his life of the long-term effects of his disease. His reaction to the disease has been to ignore physical problems and avoid contact with physicians. Several years ago he broke his finger and absolutely refused medical attention; the finger healed incorrectly.

Since admission to the facility, his weight has gone from 160 pounds to 184 pounds, which is 26 percent above his normal weight range. He has refused any monitoring of his diabetes, including weight control, finger-sticks, and venipunctures. He will allow an annual physical but no blood work.

If he has a skin lesion, he will not report it. Staff must be very astute during the times he allows showering to notice his skin condition. When

TABLE 6.1
Possible Effects of Self-Neglecting Behaviors on Service Provision

Required Provisions	*Possible Self-Neglecting Behavior*	*Consequences of Behavior*
Clean, safe environment	Hoarding, spitting	Later, overeating, overdosing on medication. Stored food may spoil and cause illness if eaten or attract insects or mice.
Provisions of nutritionally balanced meals	Overeating, refusing to eat	Weight gain, extreme weight loss, and possible starvation
Proper hygiene	Not bathing	Skin damages, body odor, health threat
Medication	Refusing to take or hoarding medication	Failure to alleviate health problems, threat to life
Supervision of health care	Refusing treatment, not bringing problems to the staff's attention	See above
Financial management	Failure to use allotted money for self-care (hair, nails)	Deterioration of appearance
Security	Inviting thievery, wandering outside the nursing home	Loss of possessions, getting lost and unable to return with accompanying danger of accident, being mugged
Planned activities	Social isolation, refusing to participate	Social isolation

lesions are found, he will allow treatment, if it is given when he wants it to be given.

PROMOTING SELF-CARE

Developing meaningful interventions to prevent or modify self-neglecting behaviors within the nursing home must take into account the community and family expectations of care, the new resident's sense of personal crises with impending relocation, and the institutional disequilibrium brought about by unmet financial needs.

Promoting Self-Care at Admission

In order to lessen feelings of powerlessness and loss of control, the older adult must be included in the decision to enter a nursing home within the limits of often highly restricted time frames (Mercer and Kane, 1979). If possible, the older adult should visit nursing homes with the family members. In most cases, because of illness, this is not possible. As an alternative, a family member should visit nursing homes, take pictures, and obtain information about services, costs, and staffing. A discussion of each home should be held with the older adult. The decision then becomes a joint decision.

An integral part of the move to a nursing home is disposing of household goods if the individual has resided in his own home or apartment. If the move into a nursing home must be done within a short period of time, much of this can be left until after placement has been obtained and the individual has had a chance to become somewhat accustomed to the nursing home. The individual can then participate in deciding which items to retain, who should get the items that cannot be kept, and what additional items can be taken to the nursing home. Individuals should be allowed and encouraged to bring as many personal mementos as possible into the nursing home to provide a familiar and secure environment. Such active measures help the individual preserve self-esteem and reinforce personal responsibility for the care that will be received.

In the admission process, the staff should direct questions to the older adult. Input on needs, wants, desires, and background should be obtained from the older adult, if appropriate. Preferences on meal times, food selection, and daily schedules should be discussed. An explanation of what life is like in a nursing home will help equip the person to adapt more effectively to coming changes. An orientation to the total building assists the resident in becoming familiar with the new "home."

Promoting Self-Care for the Resident

One goal of an institution is to provide services to large numbers of people as efficiently as possible. However, efficiency often has fairly strict parameters and limited flexibility to allow for individual difference. This system, in the name of efficiency, may rob a person of individuality, sense of personal control, privacy, and responsibility. To avoid this, the nursing home staff must be creative in looking for ways to balance required efficiency and the personal needs of the residents. In some cases, we are talking about very subtle differences in the way the nursing home staff handle everyday care needs (Rosendahl and Ross, 1982). An example might be Mrs. C, who is being informed by nursing staff of the shower schedule. One approach is to tell Mrs. C she has to take her showers on Tuesdays and Thursdays at 10:00 a.m. A more effective approach would be to state that showers are given on Tuesdays and Thursdays of each week and to ask Mrs. C when she would like to bathe. In this way, the individual has participated in the planning of day-to-day activities.

An even more important issue is choice of a room at the nursing home. This is minimized if the resident can afford a private room, which is seldom the case. Most residents find themselves cramped into living quarters with a stranger. Due to problems of bed availability at the time of admission, there is limited choice of roommate for the person moving in and for the person already in the room. The level of care needs at admission or at a later time may also dictate room assignment. However, limited choice does not mean no choice. In some circumstances, the resident may be able to choose a roommate. Other choices do exist in terms of what time the new person is to move in, what side of the room is desired, and whether the new resident would like to have the current resident present or away during moving in (Mirotznik and Ruskin, 1984). Introduction of the projected scheduled roommates is extremely helpful. Thus, although the person has a limited decision about living with someone, there is some control over the situation. If this format were used in each of the individualized activities, the individual's feelings of personal control would be enhanced.

A person's family life does not end with institutionalization (Brody, 1985). In some sense, it becomes even more important. The nursing home residents' social contacts help validate their sense of accomplishment, provide stabilization through continuation of a family unit, assist in finding solutions to problems through the maze of institutional red tape, and prove that they are still loved. Oftentimes, well-meaning families will contribute to the problems of self-neglect through the expression of their love seeing their 90-year-old parent struggle slowly down a long hallway with a walker when a wheelchair is so much easier. In reality, the prevention of the complications that come due to inactivity, for example, incontinence and contractures, is far more important than the slow, laborious walking.

In U.S. society, food is also an expression of caring. A visit to an elderly family member in a nursing home, who is slowly declining, is quite difficult. Many family members use food as a medium for setting the visit as a social occasion and a vehicle for conversation. Although it is a useful tool when used appropriately, oftentimes it can contribute to the resident's self-neglect and result in a more rapid decline in health. For example, additional caloric intake to a diabetic can result in varied complications. Fast food laden with salt, which seems to be the new rage, can be fatal to someone with hypertension.

These situations support the needs for explanation to family members on every prescribed plan of care for the resident and the repercussions should the plan not be followed. Also important is providing the family members with substitute ways to still provide care and warmth to the resident. For instance, in the case of the diabetic, either substituting one of the daily meals or providing an appropriate exchange could accomplish the same results.

In addition to family members, all planning for care provided in the nursing home should include both nursing home staff and the resident. Even if the resident has been judged incompetent, he or she should be part of this process although participation may be more limited. Preserving the resident's right of control over treatment is especially important for someone who has, through illness, lost much control over his or her life (Mirotznik and Ruskin, 1984).

Failure of nursing home staff to include the resident can contribute to a cycle toward self-neglect (Berkowitz, Waxman, and Yaffe, 1988). Yet, nursing home staff may do just that. The elder upon entering the nursing home, even though he or she may realize the need, seldom does so without feeling the loss of accustomed self-determination and his or her own routine. If the elder cannot participate, the feelings of powerlessness and hopelessness that may quite routinely accompany moving into a nursing home will develop further. Untrained staff may find it easier, more efficient, and appropriate to do tasks rather than to encourage residents to provide self-care or to help them learn how to meet personal needs within the nursing home (Kahana and Kiyak, 1984).

Thus it is most important to provide in-service training to all nursing home staff to

> sensitize staff to the problems of self-neglect and how their interaction with residents can exacerbate self-care deficits;
> educate staff on signs of self-neglect;

help staff understand that in the long run their workload can be reduced by residents who are allowed and encouraged to provide as much self-care as possible; and

provide training on how to deter or minimize these behaviors.

In some areas, group decision making may be more appropriate and effective. This includes areas with broad facility-wide application, such as meals or recreational activities. Individuals may be appointed to represent residents in various areas in planning these functions. Again, this group of residents should be presented with limiting parameters and areas of flexibility within the parameters. For example, a resident council, composed of elected representatives, could meet on a monthly basis. Subcommittees could be developed to meet with particular department heads on appropriate subjects, such as meeting with the dietitian to plan and review the next month's menu.

Meal planning can be approached in various ways. Perhaps the menus are preplanned, and the residents' responsibility is to choose what day they wish to have which meal. Another alternative is to have the list of possible soups, entrees, salads, and desserts and have the residents put the combinations together. Institutions may object to these procedures because of the time involved, but involvement of residents' planning lessens criticism of meals and should decrease the number of complaints over food service and result in a time savings. This activity of the residents has the further benefit of maintaining alertness, maximizing awareness of the environment, enhancing a sense of purpose, and developing a sense of community.

Another critical issue is the need for privacy. This includes privacy of financial matters, family, environment, and personal contacts. Most nursing homes are designed for maximum use of all spaces. Most residents' rooms are designed to meet the minimum state requirements and may house two to four people. Privacy is provided in these rooms through a draw curtain, which can enclose the bed area. The wash basin is usually located in the rooms in an area that can easily be shared, thus reducing the ability to clean oneself in private. In most facilities, staff are instructed to knock on the door to the room before entering. What often happens, however, is that the staff person will knock and then enter the resident's room without waiting for permission to enter. All staff should be sensitized to this important need.

Shower or bathing facilities are frequently off the main corridor in the nursing home. This, at times, results in older adults sitting in hallways, in shower chairs with a bath towel wrapped around them waiting their turns, or possibly being showered in one stall while someone else is being showered in the next. It is embarrassing enough to require bathing assistance, without also being viewed by all who pass in the hallways.

Much of this loss of privacy could be minimized by bringing residents directly from their rooms to the shower rooms and by using movable screens in bathing areas. A major component in maintaining the residents' privacy would appear to lie with development of staff sensitivity to the issue of privacy of person, with strict confidentiality of all personal matters, and with setting aside some area to be used by the residents for visiting privately with family.

Many of these suggestions are important in preventing self-neglect. They can be seen as ways to enhance motivation to self-care by enhancing the general quality of life in the institution. Oftentimes, however, one must respond more specifically to individual self-neglect that occurs in spite of both opportunity and encouragement within the nursing home to provide independent self-care.

For the individual who is motivated but not able (because of cognitive deficits) to remember self-care regimens, a most effective approach might be a behavioral strategy including

> defining the desired behavior,
> setting and using a schedule,
> arranging for a support person to prompt desired behavior,
> allowing adequate time for the resident to complete behavior at his or her own pace,
> praising appropriate behavior,
> providing assistance if the behavior cannot be completed, and
> ignoring inappropriate behavior; do not provide attention for complaining, arguing, or delaying. (Pinkston and Linsk, 1984, p. 65)

Table 6.2 illustrates staff responses to several specific problems.

One needs to understand why an individual is unmotivated. If staff or other mental health referral sources are available, consultation is appropriate. Without this, one must rely on whatever enrichment the staff and family can bring to the person's life. Enrichment may be in the form of continued pastoral visits if the person belongs to any religious denomination, visits by family or through volunteer programs, and use of pet visits.

In some cases, the resident may be unreachable, and we are then left with the only course possible, with staff providing mandated monitoring of health needs.

TABLE 6.2
Approaches to Decrease Problem Behavior

Problem/Need	Goal	Approach	Staff Assigned
Diabetic & snacks on candy and other snacks	Resident to snack on dietetic snacks only for next 3 months	Inform resident of importance of diet. Ask staff to watch resident more closely and monitor snacking	NS
Verbally abusive to residents in dining room 1–2 times weekly	Eliminate outbursts within next 3 months	Remove from situation, provide opportunities to ventilate with staff, confront inappropriate behavior	NS/SW
Lethargy — less reading, asleep in wheelchair, weight up	Resolve problem with proper diagnostic tool within 3 months	Determine cause — possible deterioration of diabetic condition refer to doctors with plan on workup	NS
Needs assistance with ambulation due to amputation above right knee and lower back pain	Ambulate with walker for 80/90 feet with supervision x3 mos. Provide pain relief to lower back	Ambulate with walker 3x/week and hot packs to lower back when needed	PT
Occasionally verbally abusive to other residents during activities	Eliminate abusive behavior to residents without activity disruptions for 3 months	Apologize to residents with RT present Ask resident to leave activities if behavior persists	RT
Approximately 26 pounds overweight	Decrease weight by 6 lbs. in next 3 months	Provide 1,600 ADA diet Educate resident on importance of nutritional compliance	FS

CONCLUSION

Because the nursing home is ultimately responsible for personal care of all residents, the degree to which it can successfully increase self-care among the residents will reduce the need for staff to provide such care.

The key to promoting better self-care is to understand the residents' motivation to provide self-care and how that can be enhanced. For some residents, in good nursing homes, life may have unexplored richness. There are friends to talk with, social activities that can be enjoyed, and connections to maintain with outside family, friends, and social and religious institutions. For those who continue a spiritual reverence for life regardless of its trials, or maybe even because of them, continuance of well-being becomes almost a duty. This time may be seen as a time to complete one's purpose in life or perhaps to better understand that purpose. For others, life is precious in itself in a personal way, and there is a desire to hold and enjoy every moment. Without the belief that rewarding life is possible, the resident has little motivation to continue self-care, and the nursing home staff may not have the will to promote its possibility.

The financial pressure on nursing homes — brought about by new residents who are increasingly less able and thus need more nursing care and the declining financial support available through Medicaid — may lead to a deemphasis of psychosocial care. This could mean decreased attention to behavior and needs that underlie self-neglect and erode the ability of nursing homes to upgrade training for direct care staff. It will be a challenge to convince managers that meeting psychosocial needs is the key to gaining residents' cooperation in their care and, in the long run, will lead to more efficient management.

7

Older Developmentally Disabled Adults and Self-Neglect

Allene M. Jackson and Cynthia Compton

This chapter discusses issues of self-neglect among aging adults with developmental disabilities, specifically those with mild and moderate levels of mental retardation living in the community. The authors refer to the recent literature that has begun to link the fields of developmental disabilities and gerontology and offer some understanding of the aging experiences of developmentally disabled persons. Self-neglect is a problem throughout the life span of a developmentally disabled person. Our clinical experience with self-neglect issues occurred in the process of assisting older persons to maintain themselves successfully in the community.

A variety of services and interventions is required to support community living, but this chapter concentrates on behavioral interventions that can be applied to reduce self-neglect risks. The current population of elderly developmentally disabled is defined; self-neglect issues are discussed; and behavioral interventions to reduce self-neglect are proposed. Case studies are included to demonstrate how certain conditions can be managed and what may actually assist the individual to develop new behaviors and skills that reduce self-neglect. In our conclusion we speculate about the future direction of programming for the increasing older developmentally disabled population.

AGING AMONG THE DEVELOPMENTALLY DISABLED

Professionals working with the aging population have a knowledge base of gerontology. Those working with the mentally retarded have a knowledge base of mental retardation/developmental disabilities, and those working in behavior modification know behavior therapy. Those persons that found themselves programming for older mentally retarded adults primarily learned on the job. Existing programs were modified, or new programs were created to serve the aging mentally retarded population (Seltzer and Krauss, 1987). Little cross-pollination of these specialties took place until recently when the growing older mentally retarded population forced these disciplines to learn from each other so that policies, programs, and legislative decisions can be based on common knowledge of this growing group. An increasing number of national professional organizations in aging, health, and mental retardation have recognized this need and have included sessions at national conferences and articles in their publications addressing this population. This increase in professional awareness of the population's growth and needs and the willingness to share information to develop a group of professionals with a knowledge base in aging and mental retardation are a beginning.

A developmental disability as embodied in Public Law 98–527, the Developmental Disabilities Act of 1984, is defined as follows:

A developmental disability is a severe, chronic disability of a person which

1. is attributable to a mental or physical impairment or combination of mental and physical impairments:
2. is manifested before age 22:
3. is likely to continue indefinitely:
4. results in substantial functional limitations in three or more of the following areas of major life activities:
    a. self-care,
    b. receptive and expressive language,
    c. learning,
    d. mobility,
    e. self-direction,
    f. capacity for independent living, or
    g. economic self-sufficiency; and

5. reflects the need for a combination and sequence of special, interdisciplinary, or generic care, treatment, or other services which are:
   a. of lifelong or extended duration and are
   b. individually planned and coordinated.

Although persons with autism, cerebral palsy, epilepsy, mental retardation, and a range of neurological or sensory impairments are included under the definition of developmental disability, the discussion in this chapter focuses on self-neglect and self-management issues for older adults with mild and moderate mental retardation. In looking at what constitutes self-neglect in this population, it is important to determine if it is

> inability to learn because of intellectual level, physical and mental decline, environmental and situational circumstances, or dual diagnosis;
> lack of knowledge or opportunity to learn; or
> self-neglect.

Grossman (1983) defined mild and moderate mental retardation as:

> Mild Mental Retardation, a term used to describe the degree of retardation present when intelligence test scores are 50 or 55 to approximately 70; many mildly retarded (educationable) individuals who function at this level may maintain themselves independently or semi-independently in the community.
> Moderate Mental Retardation, a term used to describe the degree of retardation when intelligence test scores range from 35 or 40 to 50 or 55; many trainable individuals function at this level; such persons usually can learn self-help, communication, social, and simple occupational skills but only limited academic or vocational skills.

Defining the age at which a mentally retarded adult becomes old is more difficult than determining an accepted definition of old age in the general population. Social Security and Medicare guidelines offer full eligibility at age 65. Qualifying for programs under the Older American Act of 1965 (PL 89–73, as amended) at age 60, membership in the American Association of Retired Persons at age 50, varying company guidelines for retirement or early retirement, and even getting a card for

Senior Citizen discounts help the general population determine when they are entering the "golden years." Although the mentally retarded population can also qualify for these same benefits when they reach the same age as the general population, they physically may have aged in relation to the general population at an earlier chronological age.

An examination of research studies and reports shows a definition of old age for the mentally retarded population to range between 40 years and 75 years (Seltzer and Krauss, 1987). Ages used by public agencies are also variable, and a survey of state developmental disabilities planning councils and state units on aging found age ranges from 55 years to 65 years (Janicki, Ackerman, and Jacobson, 1985). Reasons for the widely varying age ranges for defining old age in this population include: mentally retarded persons begin to experience decline in behavioral capacities in their fifties (Hewitt, Fenner, and Torpy, 1986; Janicki, Ackerman, and Jacobson, 1985); evidence of early physical aging and onset of Alzheimer's disease among persons with Down syndrome (Lott and Lai, 1982; Miniszek, 1983; Wisniewski and Merz, 1985); and retarded persons have historically had a shorter average life span than the general population (Eyman, et al., 1987; Richards, 1976; Tarjan, et al., 1973).

This population is very heterogeneous. Heredity, lifestyle, nutrition, and environmental factors as well as the level of retardation impact on functioning and aging. Specifically, those persons with mild or moderate mental retardation have very different social, educational, medical and functional characteristics, and service histories from those whose retardation is severe or profound (Janicki and Jacobson, 1986; Lakin, 1985), thus impacting on the aging process. In addition, mentally retarded persons who are without additional physical handicaps differ in many respects from those who have some organic basis for their retardation, who generally are more severely retarded and have multiple handicaps, and who consequently may be expected to have a shorter life expectancy (Grossman, 1983; Zigler, Balla, and Hodapp, 1984).

A common pattern of aging is not found among all mentally retarded persons (Janicki, Seltzer, and Krauss, 1987). However, there is support for using 55 years of age as the definitive for serving the aging mentally retarded population, and that age will be used for the purpose of this chapter (Jacobson, Sutton, and Janicki, 1985; Janicki, Seltzer, and Krauss, 1987; Walz, Harper, and Wilson, 1986).

Estimating the size of the elderly mentally retarded population is difficult because different researchers use various ages in their studies;

the problem of distinguishing between older retarded individuals and older individuals who are declining cognitively and functionally; the unknown and unserved portion of this population; and the lack of need to label people by disability in order to obtain services available at certain chronological ages (Janicki, Seltzer, and Krauss, 1987). Estimates of the number of persons with mental retardation, based on the 1980 census, over 55 years of age range from 472,440 to 1,417,320 (Seltzer and Krauss, 1987). In addition, the number of mentally retarded individuals needing programming, housing, and services in the next 20 to 30 years is expected to increase markedly because of longevity and size of successive generations (Janicki, 1986; OHHS, 1987). With 87 percent of those individuals with mental retardation estimated to be mildly retarded and therefore appropriate for community placement (Rose and Janicki, 1986), self-management through behavior therapy becomes more important because it can decrease self-neglecting behavior in the existing population and can be taught at an earlier age as a means of promoting successful and independent aging.

SELF-NEGLECT ISSUES

Self-neglect issues exist for both the aging and aging developmentally disabled population. Unfortunately, aging developmentally disabled individuals are at greater risk because of their disability, frequent premature aging, lack of training for independent living, aging and death of parental caregivers, and inappropriate institutionalization that can foster dependence and limited opportunity. If self-neglecting behaviors can be identified and treated, the potential for independence and a life in the community is enhanced.

The consequences of self-neglecting behaviors can impact immediately on the well-being of the individual, or they can be insidious and impact on general well-being at some future time. Examples would be the importance of self-neglect in taking medication for an acute viral infection or the immediate consequence of hospitalization and the long-term consequences on the future physical condition of a diabetic not taking proper insulin dosage and following a proper diet. In conjunction with the time factor consequences, the self-neglecting behavior itself can vary in degree of importance on total health and lifestyle and has to be prioritized for intervention and behavioral management purposes. Although several self-neglecting behaviors may be present, those involving personal safety would need to be addressed before those involving personal appearance. Following are some areas where self-neglecting behaviors can take place, with the most critical for change appearing first.

- Environmental safety issues include inability to use or noncompliance with use of stove, appliances, electricity, and sharp instruments; knowledge of traffic safety and street crossing.
- Personal safety issues include differentiating between known and trusted staff and friends and strangers who might exploit or harm; knowledge of appropriate sexual behavior and risk factors.
- Health issues include differentiation between degree of illness and seeking proper medical attention when needed; medical and medication compliance, lifestyle factors that include smoking, alcohol consumption, drug addiction, and eating disorders. There may likely be changes and/or increases in the number and degree of health issues requiring behavioral training as the developmentally disabled individual ages.
- Nutritional issues include proper diet and nutrition, including purchase of food items, meal planning, preparation, and storage; interaction of some foods with medications. There may likewise be necessary and complicated dietary changes as the frequency of nutritional management of chronic conditions such as hypertension or diabetes increases with age.
- Housing issues include finding a home in a safe area and maintaining it in a safe and clean manner.
- Employment issues include finding employment and maintaining it through proper behavior and attendance; finding appropriate employment that matches individual ability and experience.
- Personal hygiene and appearance issues include personal cleanliness and appropriate dress.

Although the preferable time of intervention would be upon discovering the self-neglecting behavior, this is not always possible. Professionals may not be consulted until the behavior deteriorates and may be either life threatening or threatening to the person's housing or vocational options. Unfortunately, the longer the self-neglecting behavior has existed, the greater the detriment to the individual, and the harder the behavior may be to change. In cases of long-term physical self-neglect, the damage from the neglect may not be reversible, but perhaps the behavior can be changed and the physical condition, which cannot be reversed, can at least be maintained.

PRECIPITATING CAUSES FOR SELF-NEGLECTING BEHAVIOR

Based on the clients that we have assisted in making the transition to independent living later in their life cycle, we believe several factors seem to place clients at greater risk of self-management problems. In establishing the living arrangements and planning the environmental and service supports needed by the clients, practitioners can address some of the following areas of concern to help prevent or minimize self-neglect.

Lack of Appropriate Role Models

The aging mentally retarded individual who is growing up in a family or institutional setting and is under the control of a caregiver can become dependent and have little opportunity to develop a strategy for good health (Delehanty, 1985), personal care, housekeeping, or social skills. Even if the caretaker promotes values of good health, nutrition, and cleanliness, individuals may not be encouraged to take responsibility for their own care and well-being and see this as someone else's responsibility. As the caregiver — often a parent or sibling — ages, is disabled, or dies, the aging mentally retarded individual is left without a source to provide needed care.

Lack of Financial Resources or Ability to Handle Their Finances

Aging mentally retarded individuals who are in the community have either been employed in sheltered workshops, competitively employed in low-paying jobs, partially or fully subsidized by family, or funded by the developmental disabilities system. Lack of their own good income, aged parents or siblings whose income has decreased with retirement, and cuts or no increase in government funding all contribute to a lack of adequate financial resources. In addition, although many individuals have the ability to learn concrete activities, such as homemaking or specific job skills, reading skills and more abstract thinking are a problem. Knowing the difference between $1 and $10, making change, and budgeting for future expenses are more difficult skills to learn and can impact on how available money is spent and on the quality of life.

Lack of Knowledge or Prior Training

The aging mentally retarded person over 55 years did not have the advantages of the mentally retarded children of today. Testing, evaluation, and programming now start at an early age, and placement in the Special School System, as well as accessing the Department of Mental Health System, allows individual skills development and access to services. Many of the aging mentally retarded persons that started in the regular school system either dropped out or were advanced because of age rather than knowledge learned. If the mentally retarded child was kept at home, preparation for living in the outside world was not considered important because placement was either home or institution. As the parents and the mentally retarded child age, role reversal can take place. Aging parents in their seventies or eighties may rely on the retarded child to maintain their own independence in the community and consider training a threat to that independence, if the adult child learns enough to live in the community.

Physical or Mental Condition

The health status of the aging mentally retarded population parallels that of other elderly individuals, with the same kinds of chronic conditions and illnesses. In addition, individuals with mental retardation are more likely to have seizure disorders and hearing problems (Jacobson, Sutton, and Janicki, 1985) as well as physical handicaps and vision impairment (Hauber, Rotegard, and Bruininks, 1985). Evaluation of cognitive functioning, dementia, and mental illness is difficult with the older mentally retarded individual. Studies of the prevalence of these problems in relation to the general population thus far are inconclusive, but these problems do exist in this population (Walz, Harper, and Wilson, 1986) and must be considered on an individual basis when dealing with self-neglecting behavior.

Environmental/Situational Conditions

The environmental conditions surrounding the aging mentally retarded individual can limit or enhance behavior. Housing, in relation to structure, safety, and neighborhood; proximity of family, neighbors, and friends; their willingness to be of assistance; transportation; and proximity of stores, churches and synagogues, and places of recreation — all impact on the person's ability to maintain control over what is possible.

IMPORTANCE AND RAMIFICATION OF PHYSICAL LOCATION OF INDIVIDUAL IN CHANGING SELF-NEGLECTING BEHAVIOR

The physical location of the individual when the self-neglecting behavior is identified and intervention is initiated can determine the individual's motivation in changing behavior, the structure of behavior therapy, and the potential of behavioral changes to decrease self-neglect. The physical location may include the following living situations.

Living at Home with a Family Member

The family member may be a parent, sibling, or other related family member. In this situation the motivation for seeking intervention and the success of this intervention can be greatly determined by the family member's perception of the problem, the need for the individual to remain at home, and the willingness for the individual to become more independent. An older parent or sibling may have great need of the assistance provided by the mentally retarded individual. If that individual were to change self-neglecting behavior, become more independent, and move out, the independence of the parent or sibling could be threatened. The family member may well undermine the training or allow the self-neglecting behavior to persist. Conversely, if family members support intervention and independence, they are a great motivator and reinforcer for behavior change and increased independence.

Living in Foster Home, Boarding Home, Shared Housing, or Group Home

Staff working with the individual living outside a family setting will usually be motivated to decrease self-neglecting behaviors and increase behaviors that will enhance independence and decrease the need for staff intervention. In addition, staff are more likely to know how to access services, can positively reward changes in behavior, and create a climate where intervention and behavior change has a good chance of success.

Living Independently in the Community

Some aging mentally retarded individuals will remain living independently in the family home after the parents are deceased, with the support of family and neighbors, or they may be able to support themselves in an apartment or home. Their self-neglecting behavior can be invisible and long-standing and be noticed only if a crisis occurs or if they cause a problem with the landlord or neighbors. A medical emergency because of poor nutrition, problems with medication, or lack of or noncompliance with medical assistance; poor personal hygiene or apartment cleanliness resulting in complaints by neighbors or landlord; and nonpayment of bills resulting in utilities being shut off or eviction — all can bring the invisible self-neglecting behavior to the attention of the community. If the individual is strongly motivated to remain independent in the community, he or she may be willing to change behavior and respond to community pressure for compliance to community standards.

Living on the Streets and Being Homeless

Although more mentally ill than developmentally disabled adults may be living on the streets as a result of institutional dumping, the problem does exist. Such individuals have to be street smart in order to survive and are profoundly at risk for self-neglecting behaviors. It is unlikely that any of these behaviors can be changed while the individual is on the street, and the first order of business would be to get the individual into some protective environment. At that time health issues would probably take priority.

Self-neglecting behavior can take place in any of these community settings. Identifying the behavior in whatever location it exists, determining the risk to the individual, prioritizing the need for change, and motivating for change will all impact on successful behavioral intervention. It is important to obtain an accurate social and medical history and to evaluate the existing behaviors. If the individual does not respond to the normal routine questions, the use of reminiscence (Gerfo, 1980) may be considered. It is sometimes easier and more accurate for the elderly individual to remember information by recalling events than by answering simple or complex questions.

BEHAVIOR INTERVENTION TO DECREASE SELF-NEGLECT RISK

Behavior therapy is the method of choice in training mentally retarded individuals because it is successful in increasing adaptive living skills (Bernstein, et al., 1981). Its use has not been specific to self-neglecting behaviors but has encompassed all behaviors that increase individual functioning and independence.

Bernstein et al., (1981) wrote that behavioral goals need to address functional behaviors. The trainer (referring to a professionally prepared staff member with knowledge of the intervention approach) defines the function of the behavior and the various methods to achieve that function. They define functional behaviors as "those behaviors that are needed for an individual to effectively function in potential future environments, that increase independent functioning, and that are likely to be reinforced by the environment."

These are key points in developing goals for any training situation dealing with self-neglect. In addition, it is important to train for changes that are needed to eliminate or decrease self-neglecting behaviors in an individual's current environment. Many self-neglecting behaviors are critical to the individual's survival in the present as well as to future well-being. Developing a behavior training plan entails a systematic series of steps that are important to follow for effective assistance to the client.

Assessing the Living Situation

Certain basic categories come to mind when deciding what is important for an individual to be able to do for independent living. These categories include financial skills, cleaning skills, cooking and nutritional skills, shopping skills, social skills, and personal self-care skills. A number of behaviors constitute each category, and choices need to be made to achieve success in the categories. What constitutes having the financial skills to live independently can vary from person to person. Cooking and nutritional skills, like financial skills, can be achieved using different plans, depending on the individual's situation. One universal goal is eating nutritious meals. After teaching the components of a well-balanced diet, the goal is to assist someone with carrying this through and eating nutritiously, thus preventing self-neglect in this area. This can be accomplished despite varying situations and skill levels.

Some individuals have health-related needs for which they need assistance. It may be necessary to train a person to make regular doctor appointments, take medication correctly, or recognize health changes that would necessitate seeing a physician. Other people may exhibit socially unacceptable behaviors and need training to learn to use appropriate behaviors. Still others may be taken advantage of frequently and may need assertiveness training. Lonely people may be assisted with acquiring communication skills and given suggestions of groups with similar interests that they can join. A trainer must evaluate a number of factors when determining an appropriate plan.

118 / SELF-NEGLECTING ELDERS

One factor affecting training programs is time. Usually in the human services field, one does not have the luxury of an endless amount of training time for accomplishing goals. The reality is that the training time may be as limited as two hours per week per person. In order to help a person increase and maintain basic skills, a trainer must be creative in maximizing the time. Thus, assessing a person's situation and building on already existing skills becomes even more crucial when time is limited.

Goal Setting and Evaluating Existing Skills

The trainer must determine what an individual can do and what skills are needed, given the individual's situation and future plans. If a person is living independently, the trainer may be able to begin evaluation of the individual on a number of skills that are generally acknowledged as being necessary to live independently. In the meantime the trainer should ask questions, including what the individual wants to learn to do, and observe the person's behavior to determine what other skills should be evaluated.

Before the trainer can evaluate an individual on a behavior, the trainer must define the behavior in measurable and observable terms. For example, a person's goal may be to learn to use the telephone. Although this appears simplistic, opinions could vary on what constitutes successful use of a telephone. Does using a telephone mean that a person can dial a seven-digit number on a rotary phone, or does it mean that a person can use a long-distance service, which requires entering a seven-digit access code, a six-digit authorization number, an area code, a phone number, and an identification number? The trainer should define the skill in a person's training program so that others will know what was meant by using a telephone.

Writing a check is a behavioral goal that would become clear to everyone if it were written as "person can write a check to any company for any amount."

After the behavior is defined, the trainer should determine the steps necessary to perform the behavior and develop a way to measure the individual's responses. For most independent living skills, this is in the form of a checklist. This checklist can be developed by having the trainer perform the behavior and writing down all the steps necessary to complete the task. A checklist developed to measure a person's check writing skills could look like this:

Person correctly   Writes date
                   Writes to whom check is issued
                   Writes amount in numbers
                   Writes amount in words
                   Signs check

In order to evaluate whether a person can perform this skill, the trainer instructs the individual to write a check to a company for some amount. During this process, known as the baseline phase, the trainer assesses the behavior to determine its level before treatment (Martin and Pear, 1988). No hints or help is given to the person completing the check; it must be done independently. A positive or negative mark is made by each step. If a person enters the date and the company correctly and signs the check, the data would be recorded as follows:

Person correctly   Writes date   +
                   Writes to whom check is issued   +
                   Writes amount in numbers   −
                   Writes amount in words   −
                   Signs check   +

The trainer divides the number of correct responses by the total number of responses to get a baseline score, in this instance, 60 percent. This baseline score indicates what the person can do before any training is implemented and helps the trainer determine where training should begin. It is important to obtain accurate baseline data because it provides a means for determining whether the treatment program is producing a behavior change (Martin and Pear, 1988). Usually more than one baseline measure is taken on a behavior, and often these measures are taken on different days.

For check writing, the trainer instructs the individual to write checks to a number of different companies for varying amounts. This will lessen the chance that the trainer gave only amounts that the person knew. The trainer instructs the person to write check amounts such as $96.41, $23.33, and $47.01, for example, rather than easier numbers ($10.00 or $20.00) because the trainer needs to assess whether a person can write "cents" amounts.

A number of baseline measures help a trainer determine what the individual consistently does correctly. Once baseline measures are obtained, the trainer evaluates this information and determines the treatment procedure. Whenever a measure shows that a behavior can be performed correctly some of the time, it is better to train this skill than to have the individual perform it correctly only on occasion. This is especially true for behaviors concerning safety. When a person can dial "911" for emergencies in training sessions only 50 percent of the time, the trainer should not rely on that person being able to dial "911" when a real emergency happens.

The check writing example constitutes a common form of measuring behavior. A trainer defines a behavior, observes the steps necessary to complete the behavior successfully, and develops a checklist that can be used for the baseline procedures, training component, and posttreatment measures. The checklist format is easy to use; others beside the trainer can use the checklist to teach a skill. When used throughout an agency, this form ensures that all staff are defining a behavior consistently. In addition, one checklist can be used to teach many people with varying skill levels, eliminating the need to develop a new checklist for each person. One may have average baseline scores of 20 percent, another 80 percent, but the same checklist can be used, with the training beginning at different steps. Many agencies using behavior therapy to train mentally retarded individuals have developed checklists for countless independent living skills.

The checklist format is one method of recording behavior. However, the checklist format does not assess some dimensions of behavior. Bernstein et al. (1981) wrote that a trainer may want to measure five dimensions of behavior. They are frequency, duration, latency, form, and intensity. To measure the frequency in which a behavior occurs, the trainer records how many times the person did the behavior and in what time span. It is important that a record be kept of the amount of time in which the behavior was observed because the observation time may vary from session to session. When the observation time varies, the data are not comparable from session to session. For example, a person may perform a behavior six times in 60 minutes one day and six times in 30 minutes the next day. The person did not perform at the same level on both days, although each day yielded a count of six. The trainer has to convert the number to get a fair comparison. In this case, the person did 6 per hour one day and 12 per hour the next.

Measuring the duration of behavior is just recording the amount of time it took to perform the behavior. To measure latency, the trainer records the time between when the person should have started the task and the time the person did start the task. Usually the form of a behavior can be measured by a checklist format. Measuring the intensity of behavior is difficult, however, and may require machines or a number of observers who would attempt to judge the intensity of the behavior.

No matter what method is used, baseline measures are obtained until the data are stable and consistent. Foxx (1982) wrote that two questions should be answered in the affirmative before baseline recording ends: "Does the baseline adequately show the range of the behavior?" and "Is the final baseline point (number) as low or lower than the data point from the previous baseline session or day?"

After the baseline measures are obtained, the trainer writes a statement of what the person is expected to do after training is completed. This statement is the target behavior, the goal the person should achieve. It is not necessary, nor even possible at times, to expect that a person could perform a skill perfectly. The criterion level set does not always have to be 100 percent. The trainer writes the target behavior and sets the criterion level, taking into account a number of factors. What can the person do now; what did the baseline measures show? Does the person need to know 100 percent of the skill or perform it 100 percent of the time? Can a person learn all of the skill or could modifications and accommodations be made so that the person can do as much as possible independently?

For example, a target behavior could be that a person will write checks with 100 percent accuracy to any person for any amount. At the end of training the person would be able to perform this independently, regardless of the circumstances or situation. However, this is an unrealistic target behavior for a nonreader. A more appropriate target behavior for a nonreader would allow for some nonintrusive accommodation that helps ensure success and may be more specific to the individual's situation, for example, the person will write a check for the rent to the landlord with 100 percent accuracy, using a model.

CASE STUDIES

Two case examples illustrate the use of behavior therapy to effect change in self-neglecting behavior. Although self-neglecting behavior can take place in a family setting, foster home, boarding home, or group home, all are structured with family members or staff available or on call 24 hours a day. In such instances, critical self-neglecting behavior is more apt to be corrected quickly or never allowed to occur. The two case studies discuss individuals in a less restrictive and less structured environment where self-neglecting behavior can be hidden and not observed or monitored so readily. In the first case study, the individual is

122 / SELF-NEGLECTING ELDERS

living in a shared apartment, and in the second case study, the person is living independently in the community.

Case Study 1

Jan is 58 years old and living in an apartment, supporting herself with income from Social Security and a small paycheck from her sheltered workshop. She is obese and has hypertension for which she needs to take medication daily. Jan has been evaluated on a number of skills, and the results show

> Jan writes and recognizes the numbers 1–100.
> She adds and subtracts one-digit numbers only.
> She has never written a check or a money order and scored 0 percent on this.
> She stated her landlord's name.
> She copied the landlord's name from a model given to her with 100 percent accuracy.
> She stated the budget categories, but did not state the amounts needed in each category.

She was interviewed about her living situation and it was discovered that Jan pays only two bills regularly each month, her rent (which includes utilities) and her telephone bill. She never makes long-distance calls because all her relatives and friends live in her city, so her telephone bill is the same each month. She needs money each week to take a bus to work, but has missed work when she has been out of money at the end of the week. She attends a social event once a week. She purchases groceries the day after she gets her paycheck but is out of groceries by the end of each pay period. She eats peanut butter and potato chips often. Medicaid covers part of the cost of her medication, but she does not set aside any money to purchase her medication, and she runs out of it.

In order to assist Jan with increasing her financial skills, based on her immediate needs, the trainer could

  1. take her to a local savings and loan institution and have her open a savings account;
  2. telephone before opening this account to ensure that this bank uses a computer to enter bank transactions (Jan will then not have to add and subtract her deposits and withdrawals; the bank will do it);

3. assist in arranging for her Social Security check to be directly deposited in the bank each month;
4. write the landlord's name and amount of rent, and the telephone company and the amount of the telephone bill on cards for Jan and train her to copy these;
5. teach Jan to purchase and complete money orders for these bills, using models;
6. teach Jan to write withdrawal and deposit slips;
7. increase Jan's budgeting skills by having her withdraw the same amount of spending money each week;
8. instruct Jan to purchase a weekly bus pass at the bank when she withdraws money every Friday;
9. help her develop a budget where she spends the same amount each week ($10 for bus pass, $30 grocery money, $10 personal money, $10 for social outing, $3.00 set aside for medication);
10. have Jan put money in separate envelopes marked for groceries, social outings, medication, and other budget categories; and
11. teach Jan to add and subtract using a calculator.

Items 1–11 above could be included in Jan's initial training plan. Eventually other, more complex behaviors could be added to this plan as she masters these initial skills. However, when Jan can perform these skills, she will have accomplished enough to have the financial skills to continue in her current situation. This does not mean that the trainer should not continue to help Jan develop and improve other financial skills, but it is a plan that helps Jan solve her immediate needs. In addition, it gives Jan the opportunity to master these basic skills, which are the foundation for other more complex behaviors.

Case Study 2

Sandy, 62, lives in her own apartment and is employed as a dishwasher in a restaurant. She works unusual hours and has a number of expenses because she owns a car. The results of her financial evaluations are

Sandy adds and subtracts three-digit numbers with 70 percent accuracy.

She has a checking and savings account and accurately completes checks, deposit slips, and withdrawal slips.
She does not write a budget for her expenses.
She has never reconciled a monthly checking account statement and scored 0 percent on this skill.
She pays her bills without assistance.

After talking with Sandy the trainer discovered that Sandy is frequently out of money. She uses an automatic bank machine and forgets to write these withdrawals in her checkbook. She uses this machine because she cannot get to her bank during regular hours because of her work schedule. Sandy has not ever reconciled her monthly statement and did not know she was charged a monthly fee. She has been sent notices of being overdrawn at her bank but has never subtracted the bank fee charge from her account. She pays rent, utilities, car insurance, and her credit card bill (for care expenses) regularly. She belongs to some social clubs (bowling league, for example) but attends only if she has the money. She said that she enjoys going out and misses her friends when she cannot go. She telephones her friends and relatives out of town when she gets lonely.

In order to assist Sandy with increasing her financial skills, based on her immediate needs, the trainer could

1. train Sandy to increase her budgeting skills by working with her to determine her income and expenses;
2. define budget categories and assign monthly amount for each;
3. include categories for items, such as auto insurance, that she pays every quarter in her monthly budget so that she saves for these expenses monthly;
4. design a schedule for Sandy to withdraw a certain amount of money each week for personal expenses;
5. instruct Sandy to stop using the automatic bank machine;
6. assist Sandy with finding some place (for example, a grocery store) where she can write a personal check to get money when the banks are closed because she remembers to record the checks she writes;
7. teach Sandy to reconcile her monthly bank statement and to record all bank charges listed;
8. teach Sandy to use a calculator;
9. instruct Sandy to write down the amount of credit card charges she makes so that she can plan for this;

10. teach Sandy to set a timer to limit her long-distance telephone calls; and
11. train Sandy to budget for her social activities to help reduce the number of long-distance calls she makes because she is lonely.

Sandy and Jan both live independently, but their individualized plans differ substantially. Yet, if each masters her initial goals, each will have the financial skills necessary to continue living independently in her current situation.

CONCLUSION

Teaching self-management techniques to mentally retarded persons by use of behavior therapy can increase their independence and avoid self-neglect both in the aging mentally retarded population and in the younger population as they move into later life. With both the advances in health care and the increase in life expectancy in the general population, we can expect that the developmentally disabled/mentally retarded population's life expectancy will increase as well (Jacobson, Sutton, and Janicki, 1985). This increase in the number of the older mentally retarded population, coupled with the emphasis on deinstitutionalization and community placement (Jacobson, Sutton, and Janicki, 1985), magnifies the importance of teaching self-management skills. Self-neglecting behavior will not only put the older mentally retarded adult at risk in the individual community placement, whether it be independent living, with family, foster home, group home, shared housing, sheltered workshop, or day program, but will decrease their potential for normalized community integration and acceptance. If the placement fails, this may mean early or inappropriate institutionalization, which impacts on the older mentally retarded individual's quality and quantity of life. This individual can also face the double jeopardy of social stigma because of the disability and functional decline of aging or because old age can make the aging mentally retarded individual more like the nonretarded aged who have declined cognitively and functionally (Rose and Janicki, 1986). In either case, the questions arise as to which existing social service network — aging or mental retardation — should assume primary responsibility for care, who is better equipped to provide case management, who can best serve as advocate (Walz, Harper, and Wilson, 1986), and most significant politically, legislatively, and procedurally, whose money will be spent on services?

Although both the general aging population and the aging developmentally disabled population of today share many of the same social and environmental risks for self-neglecting behavior, the developmentally disabled are in double jeopardy. Generally, they have not had the family support, the educational opportunities, the knowledge of service systems, or the financial means of their counterpart in the aging population. We can hope that, as each developmentally disabled generation ages, they will become more like their aging cohorts. Although their risk of self-neglect will never disappear, the incidence may decrease as their opportunities for early intervention, better education, more community placement options, and job opportunities increase.

8

Geriatric Alcoholism and Self-Neglect

Larry Dyer

Self-neglect among some older adults is complicated by alcohol abuse. Those who are alcoholic and self-neglecting have special characteristics that place them at risk for sudden, premature death or inappropriate institutionalization. The common risk factors for the development or exacerbation of alcohol problems in later years combine with problems of self-neglect to create an atmosphere of crisis and instability that can cause rapid major changes in health status. Further, the social forces in our society that sometimes harshly judge both people with alcohol problems and self-neglecting elders can result in quick fixes that are neither in the client's best interests nor what the client, when capable of rational decision making, would want.

The interactive effects involved in elder alcoholic self-neglect present highly dangerous situations. The severity of the problem, the sufferers' reputed resistance to change their characteristics, and the potential for change make this special population, alcoholic self-neglecting elders, a particularly important group to study. This chapter discusses factors involved in completing a psychosocial risk assessment for elder alcoholic self-neglect, types and levels of intervention, on-going treatment of the alcoholic self-neglecting elder, and implications for future research and service development. However, in combining areas that have as many definitional problems as do both alcoholism and self-neglect, it is necessary first to define some essential terminology.

TOWARD A DEFINITION OF ELDER ALCOHOLIC SELF-NEGLECT

The definitional problems in the area of alcoholism have been lamented throughout the literature. Identifying elder alcoholics is difficult because retirement changes the nature of the elder's interaction with the social networks that typically bring a person's alcohol abuse to the attention of the helping professionals (Gordis, 1988). Although the amount of alcohol consumed bears a relationship to the extent of the problem, definitions that rely solely on consumption amounts fail because body weight, health status, and other physical factors influence how an elderly individual will be affected. Self-report of alcohol consumption, a problem at any age because of memory impairment caused by drinking, is even more unreliable for the elderly who may have additional memory problems (Graham, 1986). Further, the condition of increasing tolerance, a symptom of alcoholism, complicates the use of consumption amounts for definitional purposes.

Perhaps the most enduring definition was that proposed by Marty Mann, founder of the National Council on Alcoholism. For the purposes of this chapter, the operational definition of an alcohol problem will be that adopted by the National Council on Alcoholism. According to this definition, an individual has a problem with alcohol if there is a consistent problem caused by or exacerbated by alcohol in one or more of the major areas of life: familial, social/occupational, legal, financial, or health. Many older adults will not be affected in some of these areas, such as occupational or legal, because of a decreased likelihood of occupational involvement with advanced age (Williams, 1984). Family life is also frequently restricted to communications with out-of-home or out-of-town relatives, so this area of detection is less often pronounced. Finances and health, however, are particularly vulnerable areas for the older alcoholic (Gordis, 1988).

Self-neglect can also be differentially defined by various sources. Most definitions begin with the failure of the individual to provide for the basic necessities of living, including proper nutrition, shelter and clothing, social activities with others that enhance feelings of competence and self-esteem, and, especially important among older adults, health maintenance (Reed and Leonard, 1989). The stereotypic self-neglecting elder referred to as suffering from the Diogenes Syndrome frequently refuses offers of help (Clark, Mankikar, and Gray, 1975). While this may hold for the elder alcoholic self-neglecter in situations where access to continued alcohol use is threatened, frequently the older alcoholic may accept or even seek out help that will relieve the effects of alcoholic self-neglect if continued alcohol use is not an issue. This difference may in fact set up a situation in which health professionals have to make ethical judgments regarding provision of services to relieve the self-neglect versus codependent behaviors that may inadvertently extend the alcoholic career. Alternatively, in extreme cases of elderly self-neglect, the individual's freedom must often be measured against danger to self, creating situations in which the practitioner must select among some strong, freedom-restricting interventions (Thomasma, 1984).

A definition of elder alcoholic self-neglect must synthesize these two definitions in some way. However, given the definition proposed for alcohol abuse that involves at least one problem in the individual's life that is related to the use of alcohol, self-neglect would most certainly coexist at least to some degree with elder alcohol abuse. The extent to which the older alcoholic exhibits self-neglecting behaviors depends upon both the progression of the disease process and the areas affected by the alcohol use. For this discussion, elder alcoholic self-neglect involves consistent neglect of at least one major life area by the elder because of the abusive use of alcohol. This then leads to a discussion of the psychoanalysis-social risk factors for alcoholic self-neglect.

PSYCHOSOCIAL RISK ASSESSMENT

Older alcoholics have been divided, for the purposes of clinical assessment, into two groups: the early-onset alcoholic, whose drinking began in early life and continued throughout the life span, and the late-onset alcoholic, whose drinking began late in life in reaction to changes in the psychosocial aspects of aging (Atkinson, 1984). Another smaller clinical category that has been suggested is the intermittent alcoholic, whose pattern of use began early but is characterized by returns to abusive drinking throughout the life span (Williams, 1984). The nature of the clinical history of alcohol use has important implications for the types of intervention that might prove useful.

The factors that place an elder at risk for self-neglect are similar to those that place an elder at risk for late-onset alcoholism (Atkinson, et al., 1985). These shared risk factors place the older adult in greater jeopardy for developing alcoholic self-neglect problems. These can, in turn, initiate a rapid, downward spiral requiring immediate and strong interventions to prevent the rapid deterioration of the health and safety status of the older adult. These risk factors include isolation, loss and grief issues, chronic health problems, changed social status, retirement, and familial role changes.

Isolation

Changes that frequently take place during the later years encourage isolation (Williams, 1984). For example, older adults frequently live alone and are no longer employed. Although many older people remain very active socially, these activities are more easily dropped than are work or nuclear family obligations for their younger counterparts if the elder develops alcoholism. Problems with mobility and inability to drive further exacerbate the potential for isolation in the elder. This isolation, and the subsequent lack of support for self-esteem, can create a susceptibility for neglecting personal care. Isolation can likewise increase susceptibility to late-onset alcoholism or a recurrence of earlier alcohol problems that might have been in remission (Perez, 1989). Isolation can, for older adults, trigger problems with both alcoholism and self-neglect that can then reinforce the severity of each in the rapid, downward spiral of alcoholic self-neglect.

Loss and Grief

The increasing frequency with which the elderly suffer losses can add to the risk of alcoholic self-neglect (Robertson, 1989). The grief of older adults is often complicated when losses follow so closely upon each other that the elder has not processed a previous episode of grief (Conway, 1988). Examples of these losses are numerous and include not only death of a spouse but also loss of many other family members, loss of the status and activities of work, loss of mobility, gradual loss of sensory input, and loss of financial stability. The compounding nature of grief reactions leaves the elder at high risk for developing depression, which, in turn, can lead to late-onset alcoholism and subsequent self-neglect.

Chronic Health Problems

As people age, most will develop some form of chronic health problem. This change requires changes in a number of related areas (Rolland, 1987). Medication must be managed, which, if alcohol is used, can cause negative interactions. Often other life events that are normally simple become more complex, such as going to the grocery store if one has arthritis with subsequent slowed mobility or if one is unable to drive because of new disabilities.

But perhaps the greatest risk factor occurs when chronic health problems include chronic pain. The temptation to self-medicate when physical pain is constant and cannot be expected to subside is great. If this is accompanied by increased isolation, the mental preoccupation with the pain that can occur increases the risk of alcohol use to dull awareness of both chronic pain and loneliness.

Social Status

The changing status that people must accommodate as they age is frequently mentioned in the literature, but it is often underestimated. The working man or woman who has had a lifetime of experiences with other people can easily become the older homebody who is now perceived by others to have lost interests in the larger world. The older woman who has reared a family that has now left her household no longer has the status inherent in being the central figure around which a family organizes. These status losses decrease opportunities to experience positive self-esteem, which predisposes the aging individual to depression and to using alcohol to mask lowered self-esteem (Perez, 1989).

Retirement and Time Management

It is sometimes difficult for the working person to imagine that retirement can bring anything but relief from the pressures and demands of a working life. The fantasy is frequently of a time when one can engage in the activities that one puts off while maintaining these demands. However, the reality of retirement for many older people is that a large segment of their time is now open for planning. The older retiree needs to reorganize time in terms of new activities with new people, because old work friends are not interested in the new activities of retirement.

Time management and maintaining a structure in one's life are necessary to successful retirement. Without these, the older adult can easily fill empty time with alcohol use. Former proscriptions against drinking during working hours no longer apply; the lonely daytime hours go by more quickly at the neighborhood bar. For some people retirement brings both explicit role changes and more subtle emotional changes that can leave the elder at risk for both self-neglect and alcoholism. That risk may be ignored when the beginning patterns of self-neglect are considered to be mere lifestyle shifts that progress into chronic loneliness made worse through alcohol abuse.

Familial Role Changes

As people age, their family relationships change. Widowhood brings an obvious change in relationship, but adult children also change as their children mature and leave the home. The adults may tend to focus anxiously on their parents' aging and inevitable death causing them to caretake "too well" for their elders. Adult children who are uncomfortable with their own aging may enable the older alcoholic to continue abusive use because of an unwillingness to confront the situation (Serkin, 1987). The middle generation is usually the organizational center of the family and, thus, in a position of potential conflict and overextension (Duffy, 1984). They may be experiencing codependent relationships with both parents and children and may save their energy for dealing with their offspring. It is important in situations of both self-neglect and alcoholism among the elderly to look at the functional age of the older adult and compare this to the age that is attributed to them within the family system (Greene, 1986). Elders may easily be treated as older and more infirm than they are because of self-neglect and alcohol abuse.

Interrelationship of These Risk Factors

These risk factors that encourage the development of problems in both areas also have a downward, spiraling effect on the elder that can cause a dangerous and rapid descent into self-neglectful behavior. The existence of any one risk factor in itself does not necessarily predispose the elder to abusive use of alcohol; however, the combination of multiple risk factors leaves the elder at significantly higher risk for alcohol problems. The rapid descent is even more dangerous because the isolation that frequently accompanies aging, alcoholism, and self-neglectful behavior removes possible social checks on behavioral deviance that bring many younger alcoholics to treatment when the addiction is life threatening. The self-neglecting alcoholic elder frequently does not work, has no family living at home to intervene, and does not drive, which precludes becoming involved with treatment through legal sanctions such as arrest. This may prevent detecting the dangerousness of the situation until it has advanced to extremes and requires involuntary intervention.

CASE EXAMPLES

Areas of life that are most negatively affected by alcoholic self-neglect include health status, physical environment, financial security, community integration, and social networks. The following section presents case examples from each of these areas. In each case situation, the initial problem already existed, but the presence of alcoholism prevented the individual from seeking help; that is, formed the basis for the elder's self-neglect.

Reva

Reva is a 68-year-old woman who used alcohol heavily all her life. She had been accustomed to money, as her husband had left her well situated years before when he died. However, Reva's alcohol use had drained her financial security, and she now lived in public housing on Supplementary Social Income. She had a homemaker visiting her regularly who called her Adult Protection Service worker to inform him of Reva's changing mental status. Despite her drinking, she had been able to handle her financial matters for the most part; however, she was now becoming forgetful and sat most of the day on her couch staring blankly.

As her APS worker questioned her regarding her health status, it became clear that her memory had deteriorated considerably. She could not report who her doctor was or when she had last seen him. However, she insisted that she sees her doctor, and would not consent to have the APS worker arrange a medical examination. The situation continued to deteriorate as community sources were pressuring the APS worker to file for guardianship. The worker decided that, in spite of her failing memory, Reva was handling her affairs minimally functionally, so full guardianship was not justified. She had a neighbor, also reputed to be an alcoholic, pay her rent and get her groceries. Her refrigerator was consistently stocked, so he did not appear to be misusing the money. The memory loss remained the same and the pressure to file for guardianship and have Reva placed in a nursing home continued.

The case worker came by to visit one day to once again try to arrange medical care for Reva but found her perfectly alert. Her head was bandaged, but she was able to articulate and recount her story. Her friend, the suspected alcoholic, had wanted to take her to the county hospital, and she had not refused him. It was discovered there that she had an operable brain tumor. This was removed, and she regained her alertness. Although she continued to drink, she could at least care for herself. Had she not been drinking, however, she might have sought help on her own for the brain tumor. The health professionals involved, although they felt medical care was necessary, assumed the memory loss to be related to her years of drinking.

Mabel

Mabel was a 72-year-old woman with a long-standing drinking problem. She owned her home but had neglected it for years. Besides many other problems, several parts of the roof had fallen in. She continued to drink and to ignore these needed repairs. The condition of her home was of major concern to neighbors who complained about its condition but did not act to assist Mabel. She came to the attention of the network of services for older people when she was referred by the county hospital because of hypothermia. Because this was December, the hospital staff did not want her to return to her unheated home. She, nevertheless, returned home and stayed there when the weather was at all warm. When the weather became too cold, she intruded on unwelcoming neighbors.

The social worker was able in time to assist Mabel in getting into public housing. (Her home was later sold at auction.) The worker spent time talking to Mabel about her move and the expectations by the housing manager that she maintain herself and her apartment. At the time of the move, there was concern about whether she would tolerate the setting and be accepted in it. The alcoholic self-neglect had both placed her life in jeopardy with the hypothermia and caused her to lose her home to neglect, creating dependence upon a new system for her.

Helen

Helen is an 83-year-old woman who lives in her own home. She had a reasonable income derived from social security and a pension from her years of work but consistently did not pay her taxes, which were five or six years behind because she spent all her income on alcohol. The initial intervention was to help Helen develop some budgetary skills that highlighted bill payment. This proved unsuccessful because she denied both the existence of the bills and the possibility that she would lose her house. A local social service agency had annually tried to work with her to pay at least the current year's taxes to prevent foreclosure by the city. As she continued to refuse to pay her taxes, the social service agency paid the current year's taxes for her, thus preventing the foreclosure (and helping her persist in this pattern). The agency confronted her with her alcohol abuse and required that the emergency assistance with taxes be linked to some positive step such as alcohol treatment or outpatient counseling that addressed the cause for her dilemma.

Pete

Pete is a 77-year-old man who has lived alone in his home since his wife died of leukemia seven years ago. Although he had always been a heavy drinker, he began drinking to the point that he was having trouble. He had been a successful salesman, selling large equipment to firms all over the United States, and had had many friends. However, he no longer had any friends over and stayed at home, preferring to drink alone. The heavy drinking caused him to ignore treatment of his glaucoma, and he became legally blind. He came to the attention of the health-care system when he sat down in a drunken stupor and called the police because he was too weak to get up. His depression following his wife's death and his blindness caused him to isolate himself leaving him without any social checks on the increasing self-neglect.

Francis

Francis was an 82-year-old man who lived with "friends" who drank with him when he had money from his social security check. He was referred to Adult Protective Services when he entered alcohol treatment at a local hospital. Francis made arrangements to live with his sister, who was willing to cooperate with social service agencies and who would not tolerate drinking at her home. The APS worker arranged for activities and continued treatment for Francis, making necessary arrangements for transportation and new clothes.

After a very short stay at his sister's home, Francis returned to his drinking friends. He was soon drinking daily. He refused any help until he called one day when all the friends were away. He had fallen ten days before and broken his leg. His friends had ignored his pleas for help, and he lay there with the broken leg. His alcoholic self-neglect left him at extreme risk for neglect and abuse from those he had chosen for his social network system.

Each of these cases portrays an area of self-neglect that is particularly affected by the abuse of alcohol in the self-neglecting elder. In making the assessment it is often difficult to separate the cause-effect sequence of what may begin as a problem of alcohol abuse that strips away health and economic and social resources. Once the cycle is sufficiently entrenched, extensive amounts of external resources, both public and private, must be mobilized if the risks are to be lessened or removed. These cases also demonstrate the difficulties of intervention when the elderly client does not accept even the smallest implication of risk. Denial, an ever present quality of many alcoholics, also takes on implications for other self-neglect risks. The following section describes some of the intervening possibilities that are available in working with alcoholic self-neglecting elders.

INTERVENTION STRATEGIES

The professional can intervene with the self-neglecting alcoholic elder at several levels depending upon the extremity of the case situation: motivational change by the efforts of community workers, when the elder is alcoholic and self-neglecting, but neither dangerous nor incompetent; commitment, when the alcohol abuse renders the elder's behavior a danger to self or others; and guardianship, when the elder is incompetent. However, in practice, these distinctions are not nearly so clear because dangerousness to self can occur as medical neglect, and incompetence depends upon the degree and manifestations of brain damage, which is an evaluation that lacks clarity.

Motivational Change

The motivation for change has long been claimed as necessary for recovery from alcoholism. The phrase "you can't help an alcoholic until the person wants to change" has justified abandoning many alcoholics until some hoped for time in the future. Motivation is also used to explain our failure to help older self-neglecting persons who will not change. However, such reductionistic conclusions beg the question of what we as helpers need to be doing. It is the business of the helping professions to help people muster the strength to try once again to change. Kemp (1988) describes three important myths about older people and motivation: that some people are not motivated (we simply do not understand their motivation); that motivation is something that can be measured as if on a linear scale (it is a nonphysical phenomenon coming from inside the individual); and that older people are not motivated (their motives change over a lifetime and effort may diminish, but they are still motivated). The point is that we may not understand or share the motivation, but it is there in our alcoholic, self-neglecting clients.

The Johnson Institute (1987) has described a method of intervention that involves the social network of the alcoholic in trying to help the alcoholic understand the urgency of the problem. This has been successful (success being defined as bringing the alcoholic into treatment) about 50% of the time, which is a healthy record for a group of people with a reputation for lack of motivation to change. However, this process involves the rehearsing of prepared roles in which the alcoholic's friends, relatives, and coworkers describe the effects of the drinking and the consequences if the alcoholic does not seek help. This method has not been widely used with the elderly, however, so its potential capacity to increase motivation for change in this population is untried.

This method has not been used for several reasons: myths exist about the older person's ability to benefit from treatment; associated with this are the negative attitudes of many alcoholism and drug counselors regarding the elderly; the social networks are not the same for the elderly as they are for younger people; and the family frequently does not live in the home, making contact more difficult for professionals to arrange. The myth that older people do not change in response to treatment clearly does not hold up to the facts. In fact, the elderly have a slight edge on their younger counterparts for maintaining sobriety once they receive treatment (Williams, 1984; Hoffman and Harrison, 1989; Vandeputte, 1989). However, treatment providers do not necessarily share this treatment optimism. They, therefore, frequently assess the treatment potential of older clients negatively (Kola, Kosberg, and Wegner-Burch, 1980; Williams, 1984). These attitudes, coupled with the alcohol and drug treatment industry preference for clients with private insurance providers, result in inadequate attention to early intervention in elderly alcoholic self-neglect problems.

Additionally, the social networks and family structures of older people are different. Because these are necessary elements in successful early intervention, the differences need to be assessed. The social networks of younger people with alcohol problems usually center on work, religious affiliation, or community organizations. For older adults the only formal networks are typically the providers of social services such as homemakers, social workers, and visiting nurses. These workers are often untrained in substance abuse treatment and lack coordination among themselves for dealing with alcohol addiction. A system of networking is necessary to coordinate community services to help older adults with addiction problems (Blackmon, 1985). Such coordination could provide the basis for early intervention efforts among older adults.

With regard to family structure, too often providers assume that because family members are out of town they are uninvolved or uninterested (Duffy, 1984). Helping professionals need to be flexible about the use of telephones and letters to coordinate with out-of-town family (Duffy, 1986) that may desperately want some direction for intervention efforts. A renewed belief by service providers, coupled with the coordination of services and family members around motivating the client to attempt change, could bring many more alcoholic, self-neglecting elders to substance abuse treatment during the earlier stages of the disease, before the stronger, involuntary interventions that are typically used in alcoholic self-neglect situations are necessary.

Intervention in Dangerous Situations

Since alcoholic self-neglect receives such limited attention from the alcohol and drug treatment community, many elders do not come to the attention of social services until they are either a danger to themselves through active or self-neglectful behavior or a danger to others. At such times, a commitment for substance abuse can be sought in a manner similar to the process for mental health commitment. Such procedures are time consuming. Commitment can result in successful treatment; however, the involuntary nature of the intervention sets the stage for reinforcement of the very personality characteristics, denial and belligerence, that frequently mark the disease of alcoholism and render it difficult to penetrate. An entrenchment into feelings of hostility and resentment can result that may not occur with earlier intervention based on assisting the alcoholic self-neglecter to develop inner motivational strength. Thus early intervention is always preferable.

Guardianship and Conservatorship

At the point that the alcoholic, self-neglecting older person has pursued a career of active alcohol abuse that has caused brain impairment, guardianship and/or conservatorship for the individual can be sought. Guardianship is a procedure in which the court system appoints another individual or the State to oversee the affairs of the individual's life circumstances, such as medical care and location of residence or institutional placement. Conservatorship places someone else as custodian of the financial affairs of the individual (Briggs, 1983). In many states, a partial guardianship and/or conservatorship can be applied for leaving certain decision-making powers under the individual's own control (Briggs, 1983).

These interventions can be very useful and life preserving with older self-neglecting alcoholics; however, the potential for misuse needs to be constantly monitored. The biases that can arise in work with people who exhibit an alcoholic lifestyle can influence judgments regarding competence, which is usually a judgment of degree, not a clearly objective decision. Kapp (1988) discusses the need for caution in forcing services on any at-risk elder stating that it is necessary to distinguish between the client's welfare and the professional's interests. This is particularly true in working with alcoholic self-neglecting elders because of the tendency to become codependent in reaction to an alcoholic.

Frequently the older alcoholic in a crisis of self-neglect is adjudicated incompetent and placed in a nursing home but receives no substance abuse treatment because he or she is incompetent. After six months of rehabilitative care, at the time of the review of the competency hearing, the elder is found no longer legally incompetent and is returned to the community (without resources this usually means skid row) only to resume alcohol consumption and start the process again. This has created a new form of revolving door syndrome in nursing home care of the self-neglecting alcoholic. Guardianship needs to be used only when absolutely necessary with older alcoholics, and the meaning of incompetence needs to be revised in our institutions as it has been in the judicial system so that substance abuse treatment can be provided during the period of nursing home care.

Intervention during On-Going Alcohol Abuse

Many community workers, including visiting nurses, protective services workers, home health aides, and homemakers, are asked to provide services to active alcoholics. Providing services under these conditions can be distressing to both client and worker, but it can have positive benefits for the client. The case example of Reva was one where the provision of homemaker services and meals on wheels kept the alcoholism from taking a complete toll on her physical health. It is important, however, to realize the potential for codependence and be sure that the services provided are meeting needs caused by the process of aging and not meeting needs individuals could take care of for themselves if they were not drinking. For these reasons, homemakers are frequently counseled not to buy alcohol for the client or clean household things that the clients could attend to but do not because of the alcoholism. These distinctions are judgments and are often unclear. Paraprofessional staff need active support from protective services workers and nursing staff to help clarify these distinctions as well as cope with the client's anger at having limits placed. For professionals, these judgments need to be made with supervision and case discussion whenever possible to ensure ethical and effective treatment for the client within the limits of the situation.

Additionally, nursing staff and protective services workers can do certain things to ensure that the alcohol abuse is addressed. The first and most obvious is to discuss it with the client. However obvious this simple intervention might be, it is often overlooked, partly because workers are busy, do not want to elicit anger in the client, or do not think it will help. The wall of denial that separates the alcoholic from the rest of society comes down not all at once, but brick by brick over a long period of time. Often the simple mention of the problem as a problem is referred to by recovering alcoholics as the moment that they began to have to look at the destructive addiction. Second, the worker can point out connections between the alcohol abuse and other problems, such as finances or health. The alcoholic cannot easily make these connections because of the denial and the use of alcohol itself.

If financial help is needed, the worker can give the help provisionally upon the client seeking some form of treatment. If inpatient treatment is refused, perhaps four sessions with an outpatient substance abuse counselor will be tolerated. These opportunities will help clients begin to focus on the effects of the alcoholism in their lives. The worker also needs to offer hope. The most destructive thing about alcoholism is its robbery of one's belief in change. The worker can explore and have at hand the name of a treatment source and how the treatment would be financed.

It is important to work with available support networks and to increase them. It is easy to assume that an older alcoholic will never go to a senior center or adult day treatment; however, some alcoholics do not drink all day at this point in the progression of the illness. Therefore, they may be open to attending some functions during the day. Increasing the opportunities for normal behavior decreases the opportunity for abuse. The client should be cautioned about drinking at the site, and the center management should be alerted to the possibility for the sake of on-going trust in the worker and support in case the client does drink at the site. A verbal contract between the worker, client, and center should state that the client would be sent home in case of inebriation.

Using other support networks such as friends and family is important. These sources can be coordinated to provide further encouragement to consider the effects of alcohol abuse on the client's life. Often the landlord is a particularly important figure in the self-neglecting older alcoholic's life and can be motivated to set limits on the client's behavior. Finally, it is important for the worker to provide nonjudgmental assistance and to offer hope. The older alcoholic has probably tried many things, which may have worked for a while but not consistently to improve his or her life, and it is difficult to believe again in one's own actions. If the worker mirrors the clients desperation, no change is possible. Modeling belief in change and growth is necessary in order to stimulate this growth in our clients.

On-Going Treatment of Recovering Self-Neglecting Alcoholics

The on-going treatment of alcoholics is frequently called "aftercare." However, the name reveals the conceptual difficulties in defining on-going treatment in this way. This conceptualization leads to the consideration of active inpatient treatment as the primary or main treatment and of care after inpatient treatment as extra. This leads to forms of aftercare such as having the client return to groups with newly admitted inpatients in order to save staff time. The assumption is that the individual, six months or a year after treatment, is in the same developmental stage of recovery as newly admitted patients. This concept of client care could be renamed afterthought instead of aftercare.

Recent conceptualizations of alcoholism recovery have looked to incorporation of developmental models that project rapid, new life changes for the first several years and then on-going growth during recovery (Brown, 1985; Metzger, 1988). These conceptualizations can and should be applied to the older alcoholic who has suffered self-neglect as well. Upon recovery, many older alcoholics will exhibit considerable interest in resolving issues that plagued them before abstinence. In fact, without some guidance and perspective, these issues may overwhelm the client and precipitate relapse. Therefore, assistance with problem solving is of primary importance to older alcoholics in order to help them prioritize and partialize the issues of self-neglect that have plagued them in the past. Erckenbrack and Klug (1989) present a scheme of aftercare treatment that includes assistance with such issues as transportation, housing, health, and social supports. The types of solutions may vary, however, for the early-onset or the late-onset alcoholic. In housing, for example, the early-onset alcoholic may need assistance in acquiring subsidized housing, whereas the late-onset client may need help in repairing a home. Similarly, the early-onset alcoholic may need assistance in forming completely new social networks, whereas the late-onset alcoholic may need assistance in negotiating strained relationships.

Workers need to familiarize themselves with twelve-step programs to assist the older adult in gaining access to these supports. Once a worker is familiar with the support group network, he or she can conduct therapy in concert with, rather than juxtaposed to, twelve-step programs (Brown, 1985). The most important element in on-going treatment is for the therapist or worker to realize that the months and years following inpatient treatment are filled with tremendous demands at a time when the individual must traverse the developmental stages that were bypassed during active alcoholism. Such issues may be different for late-onset as opposed to early-onset alcoholics. Late-onset alcoholics may be more focused on recent losses, whereas early-onset alcoholics may be more concerned with the loss of normal life experiences and lack of family support because of lifelong alcoholism. Many years of thwarted development must take place rapidly for sobriety to take effect. This will be the case as much for the 80-year-old as it is for the 18-year-old recovering person.

IMPLICATIONS FOR FUTURE PROGRAM DEVELOPMENT

Program development issues have frequently centered on the need for elder-specific programming versus mainstreaming older alcoholics into traditional programs. Atkinson et al. (1987) find that elder-specific group treatment helps older clients stay in outpatient treatment. Robertson (1989) points out that the issues that older adults bring to treatment differ significantly from the issues of other age groups. So elder-specific programming is necessary to truly meet the needs of the older self-neglecting alcoholic. The greater the disability and sensory deprivation, the more necessary are special forms of treatment that will help the older person overcome them. However, some integrated treatment settings see older adults form special friendships with younger patients that resemble grandparent-grandchild relationships that can be important social aspects of recovery for both. Generally, it would be best to increase the number of options available to older adults so that they can chose either elder-specific or integrated treatment.

The needs of older adults who suffer both self-neglect and alcoholism have not been adequately addressed by the social service network available to older people and to people with alcoholism. This special population needs the attention of multiple systems of treatment that have not traditionally worked together. Treatments need to be developed between systems, and research needs to be planned that can determine which early interventions are most effective, so that we can prevent the need for forced treatment of the older self-neglecting alcoholic. When forced treatment must occur, systems need to be able to work together to see that the alcoholism as well as the physical needs of the older self-neglecting alcoholic are met. But even when forced treatment is not needed, systems should to be able to work together to see that the alcoholism as well as the physical needs of the client are addressed.

9

Geriatric Protective Services and Self-Neglect

Eloise Rathbone-McCuan and Marilyn C. Whalen

This chapter describes how the adult protective services system addresses the problem of elder self-neglect. The elder protection movement is a fledgling compared to the parallel child welfare campaign, which began in the 1870s with the creation of a New York state case law granting children the right to be free from unreasonable physical discipline (Schene and Ward, 1988). The term "adult protective services" is a broad description that encompasses services authorized by legislation to prevent and protect adult persons (usually defined as those 18 years and older) against abuse, neglect, and/or exploitation. Many cases presented in this text involve human situations that could be referred to adult protective services (APS). They illustrate the diversity of needs that create risks trained APS workers are prepared to assist. There is much difference in the organizational structure, resource level, and authority each state and/or its local service units have to work with cases. Information about the specific program operated by the Tennessee Department of Human Services is presented because that is the program where we have worked and consulted. Pertinent information about these services and how they may be accessed will increase the knowledge of APS as a helping intervention for self-neglecting elders.

CONSCIOUSNESS RAISING ABOUT
ELDER NEGLECT AND ABUSE ISSUES

Despite the desire to believe that conditions of the frail, poor, and isolated elderly were better in the colonial and preindustrial era than in the current postmodern era (Rathbone-McCuan; in press), historians of aging indicate that this was not true. Then as now the quality of life in old age was often directly connected to the presence or absence of financial resources that the elderly individual controlled (Woolfson, 1988). Today economic resources are not a guarantee against the risks of neglect, abuse, and exploitation.

This was learned at the first national forum held to examine the problem of elder abuse under the leadership of Representative Claude Pepper and the House Select Committee on Aging, Subcommittee on Health and Long-Term Care conducted in 1978 and again in 1984. The first hearing was a testimony of human tragedy of aged persons who had been physically and psychologically abused by social intimates, often family members. Self-neglect was hardly mentioned in the forum. It sounded less dramatic than elder physical abuse and was downplayed by the media covering the hearings.

By 1984 there was more research data to inform the subcommittee about the patterns of elder abuse even though the data had failed to yield reliable estimates of national prevalence. Detweiler (1988) points out that between 1978 and 1988 the Administration on Aging considered elder abuse a priority and awarded research and demonstration grants on elder abuse and neglect. However, problems of self-neglect did not receive much research attention at a time when elder abuse research was expanding. When neglect was addressed in the studies, there was more interest in the patterns of caregiver neglect than on the issue of self-neglect, and that pattern continues in current research.

Wolf (1988) notes critically the floundering of Congressional leaders to develop a national policy on elder abuse during the decade between 1978 and 1988. False starts were in evidence as various U.S. representatives attempted to introduce federal legislation for elder abuse. She states, "Both Reagan administration policy-makers and congressional conservatives felt that family problems such as elder abuse were more appropriately addressed by the states than the federal government. It was in this environment that elder abuse came to the national forefront. There was no strong leadership in the Senate to push legislation, and even the most committed advocates were hampered by the lack of solid research on the topic" (p. 10).

Legislative efforts at the state level were moving ahead at that time, and even in the absence of a national legislative agenda, laws were being passed that addressed the problems of abuse, neglect, and exploitation within the elderly population. According to Wolf (1988), "Although the nationwide adoption of state elder abuse legislation took somewhat longer than that for child abuse, once the issue emerged states readily acknowledged their responsibility to address it" (p. 10). There was a state-by-state implementation of legislation to confront the problems of elder abuse and neglect. Because there was a great variation in the original legislation and subsequent changes in many states, there is predictable variability in state service policies. It is the state policies that set forth the parameters of service interventions and clarify how staff are to serve clients.

Advocates for the prevention of elder abuse and protection of abused elderly are dissatisfied by the lack of federal legislation that specifically deals with elder abuse. Their position is that federal legislation and funding are needed to deal with this growing problem. State-by-state elder abuse legislation — combined with an ongoing interest in the need for a national policy supporting the development of services and a strong response system among the states — is an interest of the National Committee for the Prevention of Elder Abuse (NCPEA). This interest group formalized in 1986 into an advocacy group of professionals and organizations. Their orientation conceives the problem as another aspect of domestic violence needing the same strategic attention now provided to child and spouse abuse.

Human service administrators, supervisors and front-line workers in the aging network and other social service units, and researchers through their participation in NCPEA have increased professional and public awareness of the problem, supported better training and community education, encouraged research to build effective intervention, and established a new professional journal (*Journal of Elder Abuse and Neglect*) to advance research, practice, and policy. The National Association of Adult Protective Services Administrators (NAAPSA) was established in 1987 as a more specialized focus group that maintains very close relationships with NCPEA while examining the particular issues facing state and local programs in their attempt to improve adult protective services.

NATIONAL PERSPECTIVE ON ADULT PROTECTION AND SELF-NEGLECT

The most comprehensive national survey data available on the status of adult protective services results from the 1987 survey that was completed by the American Public Welfare Association and the National Association and State Units on Aging (NASUA/APWA, 1988) funded by a grant from the Administration on Aging. The opening statement in the final report provides an accurate summary of the vital role that state government plays in responding to the needs of vulnerable citizens through protective services. The survey approach proved very difficult for many reasons:

> There were two major categories of organizations that had the legislative mandate to provide adult protective services to older people — state units on aging and state adult protective service agencies. The structure, function, and funding of these two types of agencies varied greatly, and there were numerous state-by-state variations in the target client groups.
> Computerized record keeping systems, when these were a resource available to the agencies who were asked to return survey data, produced large amounts of information that afforded different units of analysis (for example, different ways to count processed cases or actual line staff assigned to work with cases).
> Legislative and program policies established for a public social service mission were unique in many ways to the individual state context.

Although the generalizable data gathered to describe the status of adult protective services are scant, the survey contributed several important items of information. Forty-four adult protective services agencies reported receiving 190,156 cases, and 18 state units on aging indicated receiving 17,514 reports for a total of 207,670 cases reported to both types of agencies in 51 states during 1986. Forty adult protective services agencies reported direct expenditure of $141,053,260 and 16 state units on aging reported a sum of $5,357,568 for a total of $146,410,828 given as adult protective services related expenditures for 1986. Using that expenditure figure, it was estimated that 45 percent of that money had come from Social Services Block Grant funds (general social service money that the federal government passes to states for social service delivery); 39 percent from state social service funding, 13 percent from county resources, and 4 percent each from Older Americans Act Funds and private funds (NASUA/APWA, 1988). From the data it is not possible to know what percentage of the cases reported was involved specifically with self-neglect of those 60 and older.

ADULT PROTECTIVE SERVICES AND SELF-NEGLECT

Self-neglect is the largest category of cases encountered by adult protective services agencies (Fiegener, Fiegener, and Meszaros, 1989; Round, 1985; Salend, et al., 1984). This fact was most recently documented in a survey conducted by the National Association of Adult Protective Services Administrators (NAAPSA, 1990). NAAPSA members representing the APS programs in 47 states participated in the survey. One is compelled to conclude from these above mentioned studies that the problem of elder self-neglect is one of the most pervasive and urgent problems confronting these social service programs.

Results of the NAAPSA survey indicated that self-neglect is a category of risk or condition served in 91 percent of the states responding to study questions. However, in most states self-neglect is included in the broader definition of neglect that encompasses neglect of the elder from others. By combining self and other neglect into the same category, it becomes impossible to determine quickly from records which cases are actually self-neglect if they are counted under the unspecified neglect category. Despite the problem of vague categorical definitions, over half of the states estimated that 50 percent or more of the substantiated APS cases (meaning that the problem was confirmed from information collected by the worker) were self-neglect situations. Although self-neglect is a greater risk in clients over the age of 60, it is also noted to exist as a problem among younger adults who need APS intervention.

The Emerging Definition of Elder Self-Neglect

There is no single, precise, and widely accepted definition of elder self-neglect that the APS field can apply, and self-neglect as an APS risk category is subject to much controversy. Coleman and Karp (1989) in their analysis of changing federal and state trends in APS speak to the issue of self-neglect. They suggest that many statutes refer to self-neglect as "the inability of a vulnerable adult to provide himself with services necessary for physical and mental health, the absence of which impairs or threatens the person's well-being" (p. 54). Over 50 percent of the states construct their definition of self-neglect on the bases of the adult as being incapable of performing essential self-care tasks, identification of the tasks the adult is incapable of performing, documented reasons for the adult's inability to perform the tasks, and description of the consequences of not having the tasks performed.

NAAPSA takes the position that all states should be encouraged to recognize self-neglect as a category. A definition has been developed and recommended for use in state statutes and social policies in order to provide a clearer statement of the problem and provide for the establishment of indicators of self-neglect. These steps would clarify and separate it from elder abuse as well as the broader category of neglect and contribute a direction for research and practice activities. Toward that end NAAPSA has suggested the following working definition of self-neglect:

Self-neglect is the result of an adult's inability, due to physical and/or mental impairments or diminished capacity to perform essential self-care tasks including: providing essential food, clothing, shelter, and medical care; obtaining goods and services necessary to maintain physical health, mental health, emotional well-being, and general safety; and/or managing financial affairs (NAAPSA, 1990).

Hudson (1989) points out that the term neglect is used in conjunction with children and elders, but not in relation to other life stage groups. Many definitions of neglect imply that both the very young and old can be neglected because these groups are dependent and powerless and thus unable to protect themselves. Self-neglect definitions operationalized largely through wording in APS manuals have attempted to make some clarification about the phrase "protect themselves," but the definition offered by NAAPSA anchors the definition in a self-care perspective. The population of self-neglect cases predominating in APS caseloads are not individuals who need protection from others unless conditions of abuse or neglect from other parties also occur. Neglect results from what the individual does or does not do in the process of meeting basic needs that ultimately are essential for living. We believe that the search for a standard definition of elder self-neglect is enhanced by removing the implicit or explicit association with self-protection and replacing it with an emphasis on self-care.

It has also been suggested in this text that using the research base from England would lead to separating self-neglect and self-abuse from elder abuse and neglect inflicted by others. There may be more value in defining self-inflicted neglect and abuse independently from other-inflicted abuse and neglect (Hudson, 1989). The implication that self-neglect is inflicted in a manner comparable to self-abuse (for example, intentional starvation or mutilating oneself) is also questionable. "Inflicted" implies an intentionality that is not justified from the most representative cases of self-neglect available in APS records. Quinn and Tomita (1986) have defined careful distinctions among these conditions, and their work has helped practitioners clarify the complex risks present in cases where self and other sources of abuse and neglect are present.

The development of a definition of self-neglect should begin with a focus on the human needs that are going unmet, the reasons that needs are not being met, and the problems that are thereby created. An important elaboration of a needs-based definition of self-neglect encompasses the rights and responsibilities of individuals within the service provision framework. The ultimate definitions of client and practitioner rights and responsibilities will be interpreted by the courts, but a practice definition should include attention to both needs and rights.

The Emerging Intervention Approaches Appropriate for Elder Self-Neglect

There is a need to develop techniques that can assist in assessing cases of self-neglect. The design of techniques that would be applicable to APS programs are of paramount importance. Other agencies will also benefit from better assessment tools and trained practitioners to identify cases that qualify as a mandated referral or seem to be appropriate for further APS assessment. Fiegener, Fiegener, and Meszaros (1989) report that other agencies besides APS programs encounter self-neglect cases among the elderly client group. Hospital social services, home health agencies, hospital emergency rooms, and other crisis centers, such as those operated by mental health agencies, are going to continue to see geriatric self-neglect cases. Even though mandated reporting laws may direct referrals to APS, there continues to be an unknown number of cases that enter the formal system through these other agencies. Sometimes these agencies can meet needs involving the protective services system; in other cases they must proceed to make an APS referral.

Assessment must begin with the ability to describe and verify that there is a condition of serious illness, injury, impairment, debilitation, and/or endangerment. The concept of "risk conditions" seems to encompass this definitional array. In the majority of cases, multiple risk conditions exist that are attributable to some physical and/or mental impairment.

For example, uncontrolled diabetes can be associated with a visual impairment resulting from another related condition of glaucoma. These conditions have contributed to debilitation through severe malnourishment that so weakens the elder as to increase the number of falls leaving the person more immobile or unable to reach help. Endangerment is increased because the person lives alone in the daily living space. Physical impairments have created these risk conditions, and the elderly person has been unable to meet minimum nutritional standards, obtain basic medical care, and provide safe shelter accommodating increased frailty and immobility. No informal network exists to provide daily assistance, and formal services have not been accessed. Had the elder pursued medical care, it probably would have been denied because the person had not been determined as eligible for Medicaid. Neither would the elder be able to pay for emergency medical treatment if it had been required at the time of actual care. These qualities, if existing and documented, provide a profile of a self-neglecting elder client.

Evaluating capacity is a critical step in the process of planning service strategies for many self-neglecting elders because physical and/or mental impairment does impact on the client's decision-making process. Kapp (1990) reviews the extensive and growing literature on questions and techniques of defining and determining decision-making capacities. As Vickers points out earlier in this book, psychiatry has long carried the responsibility for determining mental competencies (Baker, 1989), and increasingly it shares that function with psychologists, who have produced many of the most recent advancements in cognitive assessment. Kapp (1990) reviewing some of the major critiques of decision-making assessment (Farnsworth, 1989; Appelbaum and Grisso, 1988) mentions four client-function areas of concern: is the patient able to evidence and communicate a choice and one that is stable enough over time to permit its effectuation; can the patient understand relevant information, both in terms of specific facts and the patient's own role in the decision-making process; what is the quality of the patient's thinking process; and does the patient appreciate the nature of his situation and the consequences of the decision (p. 17)? Because of questions about their validity and reliable application, standardized testing methods have limitations; however, there is increasing intent to use these instruments (for example the Wechsler Adult Intelligence Scale and Wechsler Memory Scale) for patient assessment to meet clinical standards (Baker, 1989) and legal requirements. Although medical and psychiatric input is valuable, standardized testing procedures are often not required to complete an adequate assessment of risk and needs as it is conducted by APS staff.

ELDER SELF-NEGLECT ISSUES IN TENNESSEE APS

States have undertaken different approaches for trying to gain more working knowledge about elder self-neglect within the specific context of APS service delivery. Although resources to do research are all too meager — given the complexity of conceptualization, measurement, and analysis — those states that have attempted to study the needs of self-neglect cases are advancing their knowledge base. Information from and collected within the Tennessee Department of Human Services is used as an illustration of some of the important aspects of adult protective services that also exist in the programs offered by other states.

Data Collected from Surveys and Record Review

For several years the agency has estimated that 50 percent of all referrals to APS are attributable to self-neglect among adult clients. Of those cases determined upon investigation to be valid for protective services, approximately 70 percent are self-neglect. Information contributed from front-line staff often documents examples of aged clients who are aware of their problems. On the one hand, when APS workers become trusted helpers, the clients are often willing to accept some services to reduce the risk to themselves. Workers find considerable satisfaction in being able to assist these clients. On the other hand, many clients need help but refuse it, and this becomes a source of worker frustration. As Arthur (1990) notes it is typical that self-neglecting clients are caught in the midst of complex interlocking events that are difficult to resolve. Clients may be attempting to manage daily problems of self-maintenance and/or financial management that go beyond their capacity. However, by law clients keep the authority to make their own decisions about accepting service unless a court authorized intervention is granted to APS, another agency, or individual.

The average age of adult protective services is gradually increasing so that the concept of "elder self-neglect" is an appropriate one for many APS clients who have a mean age of 67; three-fourths fall between the ages of 60 and 90 years old. Age cannot be considered a direct causal factor of self-neglect, but for those who have lived long and now experience physical impairment or the combination of physical and mental disability, without adequate formal and/or informal supports, self-neglect is a risk. The risk may not always occur because the elder is isolated or lacking someone to help with important tasks. Sometimes there are people in the informal network — family, friends, or neighbors — who are willing to offer various types of assistance, but the elder does not accept the assistance and cannot be convinced to reconsider.

From a service provision viewpoint, it is important to consider how workers initiate their client contact and interact with clients to draw them into the decision-making process. Arthur (1990), reporting on a sample of 203 randomly selected case records, notes that few clients were reported as resistant compared to those that workers considered to be either fully cooperative or totally refusing services offered by the worker. Home delivered meals, homemaker services, visiting nurses, and transportation and escort assistance are some of the resources that APS workers most frequently help arrange to reduce self-neglect risks. These services usually require some decision making on the part of the client and worker before they can be made available. Whenever possible the client makes the decisions independently, or they collaborate in decision making. Other cases rely on members of the client's informal network for decision making without shifting to involuntary measures.

The length of time it takes to get services to the client depends on many factors. Time taken by the worker to process the necessary requests may take only a short time, yet the client frequently faces a waiting period because there are too few resources compared to the need. Also, time-consuming processing may be required by other agencies that actually control access to the services APS requests for clients.

A Practice Philosophy of Adult Protection Services

During a period of increasing caseloads, attributed in part to increasing public awareness and the advent of mandatory reporting laws (Fredriksen, 1989) and fiscal crises and program reallocations, the basic philosophy of APS services could be reduced to a position of secondary importance. However, such a loss of philosophical perspective would probably reduce the effectiveness of services. Drifting from the value base of client practice could shift the worker from trying to help the client maintain control of the situation or to assume more personal responsibility in order for the agency to provide needed services in an efficient manner. Effective training, good supervision, clear and workable interagency service agreements, and strong worker peer support are factors that help practitioners incorporate the values of practice into daily work with clients.

Although no single philosophy is adopted by all APS units throughout the country, some general philosophical tenets direct the provision of adult protective services. Common characteristics in the philosophical position include the following areas: services are provided to assure that what is defined as dangerous circumstances likely to produce harm to self are minimized, but the best possible living conditions are not assured; services are drawn to prevent interference with a chosen lifestyle; and intervention initiated by the state that is not accepted by the elder and limits personal freedom only occurs with specific authority from the court.

Specific statements in the Tennessee philosophy help in understanding the approach practitioners take with clients. The elder must be involved in deciding what plans will be made and which actions are to be taken that will offer needed assistance. Clients cannot be routinely forced to accept protective services. If they lack the capacity to consent to needed services, then court authority may be pursued. All intervention must offer the least possible encroachment on personal freedom. If legal action involving a loss of rights of self-determination takes place, those rights are restored as soon as the elder has regained the capacity to make those decisions. The worker is focused on offering an adequate level of care as opposed to optimal care because the intention is to reduce risks through providing for basic needs. Major effort is made to help the client remain at home or in the community so long as the condition warrants this residence, and informal and community resources are used whenever possible to support life in the community according to the wishes of the client. From this service philosophy emerges the policy and practice directives defining the social service function.

Key Steps in Providing Social Intervention

Intervention begins when a referral is made to APS by individuals and professionals who recognize that an elder is at risk from the inability to provide self-care or obtain services. The services of APS are sought based on an intention of seeking some help for the elder. The purpose of the conversation between the intake contact and the referral source is to provide the information needed to determine if the situation warrants an assessment/investigation. In providing data about potential self-neglect, the referring person must describe the nature and extent of the elder's condition and situation.

The referring person is asked to give the elder's name and any other information that may be helpful in establishing the nature of risks and needs, as well as the urgency of the situation. Some information is requested that enables the worker to expedite the provision of services when the client is found to be in a crisis. For example, describing the elder's condition as being without any heat during a winter storm and unable to move from the dwelling would suggest a possible immediate need. A worker's responsibility is often greatly facilitated if the name of the elder's physician can be provided in the event the elder is found to be very ill and unable to give that information. Only after completing this information-gathering conversation will a decision be made as to whether the referral meets the criteria of the law regarding the appropriateness of an APS contact.

If the report is accepted for further APS follow-up, contact will be made with the elder to determine the situation, conditions, and need for services. Interviewing and observational skills work together to communicate with the elder the reason for the visit; to determine the elder's perceptions of what is needed in view of the level of self-care; and to note the elder's abilities, verbal skills, cognitive orientation, general mobility, personal hygiene, and nutritional condition. In some situations the referring person may be asked to assist in gaining access to or communicating with the elder. The referral source may also be willing to help implement needed assistance or identify others who may be willing to provide some assistance or support.

Because of the high likelihood of medical impairments and the potential need for immediate medical care, the medical community becomes a critical source of information for assessing risks and may need to be contacted repeatedly in order to gain complete information. The degree of urgency will determine how quickly services are initiated. If emergency action is needed, the full assessment may be completed after the emergency services are initiated. Needed help is not delayed in order to complete the paper work. However, the initiation of services prematurely is discouraged and believed to be potentially harmful to an adult trying to maintain independence. In nonemergency situations the time spent by the worker with the client is an opportunity to determine the client's strengths, extent of self-care, and what should be supplemented or performed with the assistance of others. If services are needed, the level, frequency, and type of intervention is specified, beginning with activities the client may perform independently. Activities required from the informal and formal systems are also indentified along with the services to be offered by APS staff. The client helps make the plan and has an ongoing role in its implementation and changes.

The Legal Aspects of Intervention

One of the nationwide myths that surround adult protective services is that workers have the state-authorized right to "control, remove, and/or institutionalize." Adult protective service programs have two aspects. One is delivery of coordinated services for the client's special, personal, social, and economic needs; the other is the legal authority to intervene (Potter and Jameton, 1986). Legal authority, far more than service delivery responsibility, is a fundamental and ongoing debate in the provision of services to elder self-neglecting clients.

Tennessee, like most other states, has trained workers to implement specific guidelines to determine when a client's ability to make decisions is questionable and contributing to serious threats to health and safety. Coleman and Karp (1989) state, "When workers use methods suggested in manuals to identify cases, such as self-neglect cases, they need to take extra caution. Sometimes, competent elderly clients make decisions that would not be acceptable to the majority of society but would be tolerated in the case of a younger person" (pp. 54–55). One way to help avoid the concerns expressed by Coleman and Karp is to use a risk-based system to evaluate the risk regardless of the individual's age.

If the elder does not consent or withdraws consent, APS services are terminated unless the agency determines the client lacks the capacity to consent while in need of protective services. Only at that point may authority be sought from the court to deliver needed services. A complete understanding of the client's condition and resources must be obtained before legal authority is pursued. Even then the goal of legal intervention must give priority to the least restrictive level than ensures client protection, and the client's condition must guide the nature of the legal action. The Tennessee Department of Human Services has a separate legal services division, and all legal action initiated by Adult Protective Services requires the involvement of a TDHS attorney. Any legal action requires that the worker, supervisor, and attorney have made the decision to pursue legal action (Tennessee, 1986).

One of the least intrusive court-authorized actions is a physical or mental examination, and both can be extremely important for elder self-neglect cases. The court-ordered examination has a clear purpose — to determine the risks to the elder and the need to petition for an order for placement, treatment, or some other services. The provision is not used unless there is a factual basis from which to question the client's capacity to consent or unless there is reason to believe the elder may be in imminent danger of death, but the information available is inadequate to evaluate the risk to the client or to petition the court to consent to placement, treatment, or other services. This provision in the law is used to obtain additional professional assessment/evaluation about the client's abilities or condition (Tennessee, 1986).

The petition will, if granted, only approve the completion of the examination; no placement can result without additional court authorization. The orders granted by the court are of two types: one requires the elder to be examined by a licensed professional appropriate to complete the physical or mental examination, and the other may be granted by affidavit or sworn testimony without the elder receiving notice or being present. For this second type of order to be approved, there must be cause to believe that the adult is in imminent danger of death and that delaying the hearing would be likely to substantially decrease the elder's chances of survival (Tennessee, 1986).

Emergency court orders may also be obtained by APS under the same general conditions that prevail for the court-ordered examination, that is, the elder lacks the capacity to consent to the needed service and is in imminent danger of death without the service. A legal definition of "capacity to consent" specifies that a client's decision to refuse services is not sufficient as the only evidence for determining the client lacks capacity to consent. Distinction is made between capacity and sanity. There is recognition that capacity may vary from one area of life to another and that the decision made by the elder need not conform to what others necessarily consider reasonable, yet it must show comprehension of the actual condition and the impact of the decisions made (Tennessee, 1986).

Other programs authorized by the Tennessee legislature provide additional resources available for adult protective service units. Accessing important resources such as the public guardianship program administered by the Tennessee Commission on Aging requires an interagency cooperative function. APS workers do not serve as temporary guardians for their clients. McKay (1984) has advanced the position that there is a need for a continuum of services to give adult protective services the appropriate range of resources to help clients. Hightower, Heckert, and Schmidt (1990) have completed analysis of some facets of the instate guardianship program to consider how Tennessee might better meet the need for a guardianship resource among nursing home patients. Strategies that afford alternatives to full guardianship are available. Limited guardianship, representative payee/legal custodian, guardian ad litem, and power of attorney provide many important options to those elders who are determined self-neglecting. These options are actually important services needed by many elderly clients even though debate continues over how these can inappropriately strip the elderly person of autonomy. These recommendations parallel the suggestions offered by Cutler and Tisdale to maintain patient rights.

Workers and Their Coordination of Multisource Services

The expertise of APS staff working with self-neglecting elders is multifaceted. Many of those who work in this area have diverse experience in public sector social services, and many are long-time residents of the communities in which their clients reside, both in urban and rural areas. The interpersonal skills they need to have and consistently apply in client interaction are very important to valuable helping, but these alone are not sufficient to make their practice effective in meeting the multidimensional service needs of clients. A significant part of the workers' time must be spent identifying, accessing, and coordinating the services that they have agreed to facilitate for a client.

Some of the agencies that control the resources appropriate to meet client needs are connected to the Tennessee Department of Human Services through interagency agreements or service contracts. These formal linkages, although very important, do not substitute for the informal working relationships that must exist and function aside from, or in spite of, the formal interorganizational relationships. Workers continue to find ways to build very useful informal connections through peer networking within the large service delivery systems.

Another skill area observed in good practice is the ability to work with family, friends, and other contacts that surround the elder in the community environment. To the extent possible, these individuals are approached as possible resources who can offer what might make the critical difference in reducing risks to clients; however, they too may have needs that the worker must respond to in order to gain their support of the elder. Sometimes key members in the family or friendship network are also elderly or have problems that make it appropriate for the worker to try to meet their needs as well. This often leads the worker to open a separate case to better enable that person in the informal network to gain strengths and resources. With supplemental support, clients may be enabled to assist each other, or other family members may be able to provide services not previously provided. For these reasons a knowledge of the family systems approach and how to link the family to the resources in the larger environment is an important aspect of practice (Rathbone-McCuan, in press).

CONCLUSION

When impaired, dependent elders are at substantial risk and their basic needs are not being met by families, friends, or the service systems, it is imperative that a formal protective system be in place. That system needs the capability to evaluate the risks and needs of the elder and develop a plan for intervention that recognizes the remaining strengths of the older person and supplements in those areas of risk that put the adult in danger. Elders do not always accept what may be the best or most complete solution to their situation, but most do allow APS staff to work with them and do accept assistance that at least lowers the level of risk. Some adults, capable of making the decisions, refuse the offer of help. A small percentage warrants legal intervention, which authorizes services, medical treatment, and/or placement without the adult's consent. Legal action should be available but never taken lightly.

We recognize that a system must be in place to respond to the needs of self-neglecting elders. We also recognize that there are many challenges ahead in efforts to protect our vulnerable elderly. It has been implied that health and mental health services have a critical role to play in self-neglect cases because of the impairments that cause the client to self-neglect. In this condition, unlike elder physical abuse, the role these professionals and systems need to play far surpasses the need to involve the law enforcement system. We see no utility and many disadvantages in applying the law enforcement model as the way to evolve more responsive adult protection services for self-neglecting cases.

The type of domestic trauma found among family systems in self-neglect cases has much to do with resources, competencies, and capacities to provide the care that the client needs. On the one hand, the orientation toward seeking family involvement in the lives of these elders is a principle of both philosophy and practicality. On the other hand, this approach may need to be reconsidered if we are asking people to assume what they cannot do without great difficulty and potential resentments. Nothing is gained if a case of elder self-neglect progresses to a case of family neglect or abuse because of caregiver burdens.

We are concerned about the professional and community perception that some elderly persons have such high dependency needs that they will go to any extremes to gain the attention of other people — family, friends, and/or potential professional helpers. The clinical literature contains reference to the belief that a pathological level of dependency can lead to drastic behaviors that include intentional self-neglect in order to fulfill some personality-based need. Although in a very small minority of cases the client's attention-seeking behaviors may take such extreme forms, no evidence suggests that this interpretation has any application to most situations of elder self-neglect.

Elderly persons do not want to be rescued. On the contrary, clients will usually resist the efforts of those who want to rescue them. One of the most frequent examples of this is the elder's resistance of accepting someone's definition of the need for placement in a protected environment. People resist help, in whatever form it might be offered, for many different reasons. Our experience suggests that accepting help might well represent a venture into an unknown situation, and very few of us willingly take steps into the unknown that may limit our freedom. An institutional placement, for example, is not an adventure to be taken by most older people as a fully voluntary step. Much clinical research is needed to better understand the degrees of voluntary choice that elderly people make in view of cultural values that support the continued right for autonomy among disabled persons.

An interdependent approach to practice, one that focuses on strengths and balances those with deficits, is now emerging in clinical gerontology. This system of practice makes it possible to transform the client's aloneness into a working partnership where the worker offers caring and demonstrates a competency to make life a little better in accordance with the client's definition of what gives a greater quality of life.

Among the greatest challenges to adult protective services will be expanding service delivery and refining intervention competencies for direct client service as programs are pressured to do more with less. Many new models of delivery, which connect the health, mental health, and legal systems into an active service partnership with adult protective services, will be required as the human need for service grows.

10

Conclusion: Research and Clinical Directions in Self-Neglect

Eloise Rathbone-McCuan and Dorothy R. Fabian

Our original interest in elder self-neglect emerged from questions being raised by case managers and adult protective services staff in their work. This book was prepared to help them and others increase practice effectiveness in many different situations where elder self-neglect seemed to be a major problem. During the earliest stages of the project we learned that practice effectiveness could not be substantially increased without focused research conducted by many disciplines in active collaboration with practitioners. The goal of our conclusion is to summarize specific issues and questions that should be the focus of applied research and experimental programs enhanced by rigorous evaluation.

BROADENING THE INTEREST IN GERIATRIC SELF-CARE

Material on the subject had not been brought together before, so it was inevitable that we would need to rely on other concepts to gain further understanding of the phenomenon of elder self-neglect. Throughout several of the chapters are references to self-care. This foundation concept, too rarely included in the clinical geriatric literature, is reflected in our society's commitment to prevent elderly people from being unnecessarily placed in institutions, to preserve their opportunities for maximum independence as long as possible, and to provide access to and facilitate the utilization of health, mental health, and social services.

Elder self-care is also at the center of many innovations devised in the 1970s and 1980s in health and social services to control costs associated with the inability of the elderly to care for their own essential life needs. These trends are also gradually forcing the mental health care system to include lower cost models of care.

Health-Oriented Self-Care Focus

The issue of self-care is vital to this country's current policies of health-care resource distribution, availability, cost and finance structure, and utilization. Citizens are being expected to engage in greater responsibility for their health maintenance, welcome the advent of outpatient care formerly provided through inpatient hospitalization, and accept, if not expect, their social support network to assist them with acute care follow-up and chronic long-term care. Shifts such as these toward greater personal responsibility have left direct care health professionals with the challenge to articulate the complex relationship between contemporary health issues and approaches to effective patient self-care (Woods, 1989).

Holstein (1986) presents an analysis of the conceptual themes that have contributed to specific definitions of self-care and their applications to geriatric health care connected to the larger societal shift of the 1970s toward "self-health." At the center of that care agenda were the self-care initiatives involving individual functions to promote personal health and more consumer-oriented responses from the primary health-care system (Levin, Katz, and Holst, 1976). The concept of self-care was quickly expanded to include the specification of behavioral aspects of professional consultation and the possible interaction between self-care and professional care. Hickey (1981) was among the first gerontologists to apply self-care behaviors to an analysis of health-care behavior of older people that includes:

- the most basic daily health maintenance behavior such as good nutrition and dental hygiene;
- the recognition and interpretation of symptoms;
- interaction with social support networks and with the health-care system, including taking an assertive role in health-care decision making;
- various forms of self-treatment;
- compliance with prescribed or other remedial efforts; and
- health education, including the application of health skills such as taking one's blood pressure or administering injections.

Kane and Kane (1986) provide a macroperspective of the self-care movement and its implications for older people: "The elderly use health care services, and their self-care must include efforts to get the most benefits and the least harm from such care. Simultaneously, work can take place on two fronts: educating health care providers to ways of fostering self-care and self-help activities in their elderly clients, and social action to try to reshape the health care delivery system" (p. 251). They make a strong case for connecting the elder self-care promotion agenda to the systems level concerns of health care and related services so as to provide coordination leading to better geriatric health care.

Hickey, Dean, and Holstein (1986) describe the broad diversity of meanings that gerontologists have ascribed to self-care. "Self-care has been used to describe a variety of phenomena ranging widely from preventive health measures as a kind of antidote for aging to enlightened consumerism, lay care, and self-help. Self-care has also been suggested as a medical care alternative" (p. 1363).

The operational definition of self-care proposed by Woods (1989) is drawn from the work of Orem (1980; 1985), who conceptualized three categories of self-care as universal, developmental, and health-deviation and introduced the concept of self-care agency into the increasingly broad typology of health-care settings. Medical sociology (Mechanic, 1960; 1968) is another theoretical source that underlies the health-oriented models of self-care framed by Woods. The broad definition Woods (1989) offers for self-care is, "A person's attempt to promote optimal health, prevent illness, detect symptoms at an early date and manage chronic illness. Self-care may also include processes of self-monitoring and assessment; symptom perception and labeling; evaluation of severity; and evaluation and selection of treatment alternatives, such as self-help, lay helping resources, or formal health services" (p. 2). To have direct application to elder self-neglect, the concept of self-care would have to be expanded beyond biological and physical symptoms and illnesses to include psychological, social, and economic needs, which are now met through personal action that draws on internal and external environmental resources beyond the boundaries of the health-care system.

From the perspective of elder self-care and self-neglect, we strongly support developments in the health and medical service fields but believe effort must not end there. The practice-based analyses of self-neglecting elderly persons included in this book give evidence of the importance of not limiting our concern for, or understanding of, self-neglect by means of the medical model framework in which compliance and adherence to therapeutic regimes are sometimes the too-narrow focus. Our desire is to see the greater availability of comprehensive resources necessary to maintain self-care capacity or transform self-neglect into self-care expanded beyond the individual to the family, community, and society as a whole. Woods (1989) also refers to the importance of including family and community systems in her health-oriented self-care model.

The Elder's Self-Care Task Performance

To meet their own needs, elderly persons must minimally apply a variety of cognitive strategies that involve the complex relationship of self to their environment; utilize physical energy and strength to accomplish activities; and rely, more or less, on resources beyond themselves when these are available and/or accepted. Upon their return from home visits, case management staff and adult protection service workers we were in contact with were expected by their agencies to have some understanding of the elders' ability to meet their own basic needs. These service providers, like many employed to care for frail elderly patients, lack specialized training that would enable them to discern the complexities of self-care task performance, a requirement to evaluate adequately the risks of self-neglect. The actual assessment of high-risk clients includes making some determination of the clients' reactions to self-care demands. As Reese and Rodeheaver (1985) point out, the study of the elderly person's performance of real-life tasks in the normal ecological environment is both complex and limited. Elder self-maintenance involves concrete situations of basic personal care requirements and some behavioral output in face of various constraints with various potentials of response. The understanding of task performance — from which much self-neglect risk occurs — is only as adequate as the information gathered. Usually only the most sophisticated clinical settings or comprehensive multiservice agencies have adequate staff and technology to do systematic observation and analyses of the processes that are associated with self-care task performance.

ASSESSMENT AS A CONTINUING PRIORITY FOR REFINEMENT

Assessment has been a major area of concern in many chapters. While different approaches, objectives, and outcomes have been emphasized by the authors, the following definition of assessment encompasses their orientations:

Assessment is the process of gathering information about an individual or group for the purpose of answering certain clinical or research questions. Four prominent objectives of assessment can be identified ... to find out whether the problems presented by a given individual meet designated criteria for inclusion in a diagnostic category ... to assess the broad patterns of behaviors, thoughts or emotions of the individual in order to provide more complete information about dimensions of current functioning than is encompassed by diagnosis ... to evaluate specific variables that can assist in treatment planning, especially in deciding among alternative forms of treatment. Finally, assessments can measure critical variables for the purpose of evaluating the outcomes of interventions (Zarit, Eiler, and Hassinger, 1985, p. 725).

Vickers considers assessment from a more traditional diagnostic perspective and discusses the spectrum of biopsycho and nutritional conditions that could cause or be critically associated with self-neglecting behaviors. However, he makes it clear that no specific diagnosis, per se, exists for self-neglect. If self-neglect is present, it will be associated with, or be a symptom of, other conditions or diseases that must be accurately diagnosed. The general framework of elder self-neglect, according to Rathbone-McCuan and Bricker-Jenkins, emphasizes that a major part of the assessment process must attend to the personal thoughts, meanings, and actions involved in the elder's self-care process.

Behavioral assessment is the foundation for constructing the self-care skills training that Jackson and Compton have found successful with developmentally disabled older persons learning to live in the community for the first time. The older alcoholic client's assessment recommended by Dyer addresses an in-community approach similar to that generally applied in cases seen by the adult protective service workers discussed by Rathbone-McCuan and Whalen.

The family systems perspective of assessment presented by Wilner and Vosler can be applied in the majority of cases where evaluation of social supports is appropriate. Hashimi and Withers illustrate the important interplay between individual and environmental interactions as a way to understand the subtle problem of self-neglect in nursing homes. A wide variety of self-report measures that assess affect and behavior as they apply to self-neglect problems have potential applications to the older population (Zarit, Eiler, and Hassinger, 1985).

Recently, gerontologists, for example, Kane (1990), recognized for their expertise in assessment, have discussed the importance of comprehensive assessment to determine the ability of elderly persons to perform and learn new skills vital for self-care:

> Self-care capacity is based on functional performance, which, is a product of the person's physical and mental capabilities, his/her psychological motivation, and the environmental pressures. Therefore, the entire physical, emotional, cognitive, and environmental assessment will yield information about the ability of the individual to sustain an independent life-style. But a more direct way of tapping into this content is to assess self-care performance directly [through activities of daily living and instrumental activities of daily living] (p. 74).

Numerous refinements in assessment have further added to the validity, reliability, and usefulness of self-care evaluation. Multiple raters have been used and scales have attained greater interrater reliability so that self-care skills may be measured more accurately. Assessments conducted in the natural environments of the elderly have become more prevalent so that unfamiliar environments do not create an artificial assessment context. Integration between the measured capacity and intervention to improve capacity is assessed as part of treatment outcome, included when measuring client benefits. Conditions under which assessments are performed are better controlled to screen out the influences of elder drug or high stress reactions. Persons with cognitive limitations are carefully evaluated to eliminate inappropriate generalizations about skill loss, and the assessment of ability with assistance from other persons and/or technologies is viewed as functional interdependence rather than quickly labeled dependent functioning and assessed as such. Cognitive functioning now relies on assessment or test results in the areas of attention, language, memory, visuospatial ability, and conceptualization, and this measurement is combined with a greater attention to the prior knowledge that the elderly person would possess and reflect in some forms of testing (Albert, 1988).

Within the past few years, settings for specialized geriatric assessment have been developed. They are increasing in number and are becoming a part of the care continuum in large teaching hospitals where geriatric medicine is an established specialty. Gallo, Reichel, and Andersen (1988) describe the interdisciplinary team as a necessary core to provide the multidimensional screening that many self-neglecting elderly greatly need but do not receive. Among the many benefits offered by these programs are the specialized assessment resources for providing dementia diagnoses, expanded supports and expertise available to the primary care physician, and opportunities for rehabilitation therapies through assessment outcomes coordinated with medical and health rehabilitation specialties.

AUTONOMY: A CENTRAL PRACTICE INTERVENTION

The chapter prepared by Cutler and Tisdale provides a detailed analysis of the many ethical issues that face practitioners and require resolution in the process of providing appropriate services. These ethical issues, once only considered within the professional codes of ethics, are becoming ever more sharply defined as the courts emerge as the authority for settling disputes and establishing judgments about protecting client rights and freedoms. Vickers considers how these legal decisions have reduced the control of psychiatrists over patients whom they once dominated in the name of client and community good. The extent to which the intervention protocols used in adult protective services are developed within the legal framework set forth by the courts to safeguard individual rights is discussed by Rathbone-McCuan and Whalen.

A significant amount of applied research on personal autonomy and long-term care has just been released from the final reports of the Personal Autonomy in Long-Term Care Initiative, a four-year, 28-project grant program sponsored by the Retirement Research Foundation (Hofland, 1990). Although none of these projects focused specifically on elder self-neglect, many programs under this initiative served at least some clients who were at possible risk of self-neglect. Some of the interconnections between the different levels of autonomy and points made in this book are summarized below:

1. Three dimensions of autonomy were identified from the projects and formed a hierarchical continuum. Physical autonomy applied to freedom of mobility, physical independence, and use of the least restrictive environment. Hashimi and Withers point out that mobility is an important quality of life factor for nursing home patients, including those with dementia who are more likely to have movement restricted. When a facility maintains an open physical environment for patients, the staffing requirements need to be appropriate to both observe and engage with patients so as to add complementary supports for increased physical mobility. Furthermore, the least restrictive environment was present as both a legal and policy requirement of serving the self-neglect cases in

Tennessee. Not all states have this emphasis, but Rathbone-McCuan and Whalen consider that workers need to incorporate a value for the least restrictive environment in their practice philosophy.

2. The psychological dimension of autonomy relates to control over one's environment and choice of options. Fabian and Rathbone-McCuan focus on the Social Breakdown Syndrome and the Diogenes Syndrome, also mentioned by Dyer, as being based on environmental choices made by persons about how they will live. However, those choices were potentially perceived by others to imply some aberrant mental condition. Wilner and Vosler identify how closed family systems, even those that provide responsible care to dependent elders, may isolate the aged person and caregiver from external supports and, as a result, increase neglect risks.

3. The spiritual dimension of autonomy is anchored in the meaning and expression of self through lifelong values and experience. Rathbone-McCuan and Bricker-Jenkins recommend that these be fully considered in the process of determining self-neglect risks, as the behavior patterns required for personal and environmental maintenance are usually anchored in value structures and important definitions of self-meaning (Hofland, 1990, pp. 5–6). In fact, many authors imply the importance of the spiritual dimension of autonomy without applying this important concept.

POSSIBLE DIRECTIONS IN ELDER SELF-NEGLECT RESEARCH

Developing an adequate knowledge base will require collecting epidemiological data that allow us to understand the distribution of self-neglect in the elder population and the factors that influence its distribution. Epidemiological methods are already being applied ever more frequently in the field of gerontology, for example, in geriatric psychiatry and public health. But other types of research on elder self-neglect are needed before meaningful prevalence and incidence studies can be conducted. The concept remains so ambiguous that observers are certain to vary widely in identifying self-neglect cases.

A theme running throughout this text is the difficulty of separating out the ubiquitous conditions of aged persons who ignore some aspect of their self-care that may create some risk from those in a serious state of self-neglect resulting from physical, mental, or combined impairments. A starting point for the future study of elder self-neglect is to gather information from samples of elderly persons in which self-neglect occurs. Authors have discussed instances of self-neglect as a problem among clients in specific subgroups of elderly. We lack the data to distinguish between individuals where there is a historical pattern to the self-neglect as compared to a late-onset pattern, but this difference would be important to explore further to understand the disability-related aspects of self-neglect in later life. It would also be relevant to investigate health, mental health, and social service utilization of elders at risk of self-neglect beyond the scope of adult protective services, which currently touch the lives of only a very small number of elderly individuals.

Case Identification as a Source of Knowledge Building

Clinicians find themselves having to distinguish self-neglect, that is, conditions placing elders at serious risk because of physical and/or mental impairment, from patterns of life-style and personal choice. An important step that clinicians must take is the continued refinement of the characteristics or criteria that separate a case from a noncase. Blazer (1989) points out that case identification is also the foundation of descriptive epidemiology because it is the numerator from which prevalence and incidence proportions are derived. The information included by some authors has been framed around purposefully selected case illustrations from their practice, but careful case reviews of large samples are needed to develop a profile(s) that further refines understanding of self-neglect risks.

The task of gathering a large number of case records for clinical analysis would be difficult, however, because of obstacles hindering the identification of appropriate records. Dyer points out that very few older alcoholics enter formal treatment programs so that it is indeed difficult to gather samples of cases that meet the age criterion of a geriatric alcoholic even though an increasing amount of attention is being given to alcohol abuse problems in later life. A similar problem of constructing case-based samples from mental health clinic records would be faced because the percentage of elderly seen in mental health centers is so small. Despite the many biases, in particular the lack of representativeness, a national randomized study based on case records is greatly needed. Advocacy for such a study of self-neglect cases served by public social service agencies is a top priority of the National Association of Adult Protective Services Administrators.

There is valuable clinical information to be gathered from investigating self-neglect as a risk condition (sometimes identified as a

170 / SELF-NEGLECTING ELDERS

specific symptom) in geriatric depression and individuals with late-onset schizophrenic symptoms. On the one hand, Christison, Christison, and Blazer (1989) note that chronic institutionalization of schizophrenic patients in the past, coupled with increased mortality, rendered community follow-up studies inadequate. On the other hand, there are many unanswered questions, some probably derived from myths and stereotypes, about the burnout patterns of schizophrenic symptoms and the deprivation of older street people, who are often assumed to be self-neglecting. Additional studies of the patterns of schizophrenia in later life would be a major contribution from the emerging field of geropsychiatry (Cohen, 1990).

Qualitative Studies to Build Knowledge

Having identified some of the barriers to applying epidemiological and record-based surveys to advance the knowledge base about elder self-neglect, we consider other research approaches that can be applied more immediately. Rowles and Reinharz (1988) have discussed some applications of qualitative methods to the study of the frail elderly. The methods possess both advantages and disadvantages but seem applicable to studies of elder self-neglect. They state

> Qualitative gerontology is concerned with describing patterns of behavior and processes of interaction, as well as revealing the meaning, values, and intentionalities that pervade elderly people's experience in relation to old age. In addition, qualitative gerontology seeks to identify patterns that underlie the life works of individuals, social groups, and larger systems as they relate to old age. . . . [Qualitative research] attempts to tap the meanings of experienced reality by presenting analyses based on empirically and theoretically grounded descriptions (p. 6).

The general framework of elder self-neglect presented by Rathbone-McCuan and Bricker-Jenkins is derived, in part, from the qualitative data gathered from in-depth interviews with elder self-neglect adult protective services clients from Tennessee. From themes that emerged through these interviews, the authors became aware of a possible pattern they refer to as adaptive comprehension. The elders saw their adjustments to both personal and environmental limitations as satisfactory so long as they allowed them the opportunity to maintain a sense of independence and personal control. The same behaviors, however, were often perceived by those in their formal and informal network as indicators of self-neglect. This "reality discrepancy" seems to be a component of the resistance to services that often makes providing assistance difficult. The methodological value and appropriateness of qualitative research warrants further consideration as a powerful research design to study elder self-neglect.

Final Thoughts on Elder Self-Neglect

From the collective contributions presented in this book, we believe that some important avenues of further exploration have been identified. Some of the areas most critical for continued attention are intended as encouragement for all the professions and disciplines that can make contributions to preventing and resolving conditions of elderly self-neglect. First, self-neglect is an individual experience that endangers the well-being, potentially the life, of older people. To find solutions to meet the human needs that give rise to and perpetuate self-neglect will require a response from many service delivery systems. The role of adult protective services in serving cases of self-neglect is clear; however, more resources are needed to expand this relatively new social service, and urgent attention needs to be given to coordinate other medical, psychiatric, social, economic, and legal resources.

Second, the social and political implications of elder self-neglect have been paid less attention than the individual experience, as it was our intention to address self-neglect in a multidisciplinary practice framework. We have found little data to inform us about the probable relationship between poverty and self-neglect and the equally powerful association between inadequate health-care availability and individual health conditions that progress into self-neglect risks. The ever expanding numbers of health and social service practitioners entering service roles to the elderly cannot be expected to be the single source of advocacy for the most at-risk subgroups of elderly. Therefore, ways must be found to place the needs of the most vulnerable at the center of the many political and social advocacy efforts continuing on behalf of and being conducted by older Americans. Elderly persons in need of the most vocal and direct advocacy have the least opportunity to voice their own needs to the political and policy decision making sectors in the United States.

A final point of concern is the extent to which informal care provided to the elderly, including the most at-risk, occurs with minimal or no ongoing professional care complement. The demographic and economic imperatives that face our society well into the next century suggest that the failure to recognize the inevitable shifts toward less informal care available for ever greater numbers of very old persons undoubtedly requires a massive restructuring of the public service sector's ability to provide nationalized systems of social services and economic support. The current trends toward proposing and requiring private solutions through profit service provision to meet public need seem destined to fail because they will not distribute life-sustaining resources to the growing numbers of people advancing into old age without the personal resources to command even a modest level of economic and social well-being. It is not adequate for our social welfare and health-care systems to respond only to the private troubles of self-neglect issues when their needs so obviously reflect the lack of commitment to resolving societal issues.

Bibliography

Albert, M. A. (1988). Assessment of cognitive dysfunction. In M. S. Albert and M. B. Moss (eds.), *Geriatric Neuropsychology*. New York: The Guilford Press (pp. 57–81).
American Psychiatric Association (1987). *Diagnostic and Statistical Manual of Mental Disorders* (3rd ed., rev.). Washington, DC: American Psychiatric Press.
Ancill, R. J., Embyry, G. D., Macewan, G. W., and Kennedy, J. S. (1988). The use and misuse of psychotropic prescribing for elderly psychiatric patients. *Canadian Journal of Psychiatry 33*: 585–98.
Anderson, R. E., and Carter, I. (1984). *Human Behavior in the Social Environment: A Social Systems Approach* (3rd ed.). New York: Aldine.
Appelbaum, P. S., and Grisso, T. (1988). Assessing patient capacity to consent to treatment. *New England Journal of Medicine 319* (25): 1935–38.
Archer, J., and Gruenberg, E. M. (1982). The chronically mentally disabled and "deinstitutionalized." *Annual Review of Public Health 3*: 445–68.
Aronson, M. K., Bennett, R., and Gurland, B. (1983). *The Acting-Out Elderly*. New York: The Haworth Press.
Arras, J. D. (1987). A philosopher's view. *Generations 11*: 65–66.
Arthur, H. F. (1990). *Self-Neglecting Adults in Tennessee*. Unpublished manuscript.
Atkinson, R. (1984). Substance use and abuse in late life. In R. Atkinson (ed.), *Alcohol and Drug Abuse in Old Age*. Washington, DC: American Psychiatric Press (pp. 2–21).
Atkinson, R., Turner, J., Kofoed, L., and Tolson, R. (1985). Early versus late onset alcoholism in older persons: Preliminary findings. *Alcoholism: Clinical and Experimental Research 9* (6): 513–15.
Baigis-Smith, J., Smith, D. A., and Newman, D. K. (1989). Managing urinary incontinence in community-residing elderly persons. *The Gerontologist 29*: 229–33.

Baker, F. M. (1989). Screening tests for cognitive impairments. *Hospital and Community Psychiatry* 40 (4): 339–40.

Bartus, R. T. (1990). Drugs to treat age-related neurodegenerative problems. *Journal of the American Geriatrics Society 38*: 680–95.

Beauchamp, T. L., and Childress, J. F. (1989). *Principles of Biomedical Ethics* (3rd ed.). New York: Oxford University Press.

Benshoff, J. J., and Robberto, K. A. (1987). Alcoholism and the elderly: Clinical issues. *Clinical Gerontology* 7: 3–14.

Berkowitz, M. W., Waxman, R., and Yaffe, L. (1988). The effects of a resident self-help model on control, social involvement, and self-esteem among the elderly. *The Gerontologist 28* (5): 620–24.

Bernstein, G. S., Ziarnik, J. P., Rudrud, E. H., and Czajkowski, L. A. (1981). *Behavioral Habilitation through Proactive Programming.* Baltimore: Paul H. Brookes.

Bertalanffy, L. Von (1968). *General Systems Theory.* New York: Braziller.

Blackmon, B. (1985). Networking community services for elderly clients with alcohol problems. In E. Freeman (ed.), *Social Work Practice with Clients Who Have Alcohol Problems.* Springfield: Charles B. Thomas (pp. 189–201).

Blazer, D. (1989). Major depression in late life. *Hospital Practice 24*: 69–79.

Blazer, D. G. (1989). The epidemiology of psychiatric disorders in late life. In E. V. Busse and D. G. Blazer (eds.), *Geriatric Psychiatry.* Washington, DC: American Psychiatric Press (pp. 235–62).

Blazer, D. G., Bachar, J. R., and Manton, K. G. (1986). Suicide in later life: Review and commentary. *Journal of the American Geriatrics Society 34*: 519–25.

Bondy, P. K. (1985). Disorders of the adrenal cortex. In J. D. Wilson and D. W. Foster (eds.), *William's Textbook of Endocrinology* (7th ed.). Philadelphia: W. B. Saunders (p. 816).

Booth, T. (1986). Institutional regimes and induced dependency in homes for the aged. *The Gerontologist 26* (4): 418–28.

Bowen, M. (1978). *Family Therapy in Clinical Practice.* New York: Aronson.

Brandon, S., and Gruenberg, E. M. (1966). Measurement of the incidence of chronic severe social breakdown syndrome. *Milbank Memorial Fund Quarterly 44* (January, Part II): 129–42.

Braun, J. V., Wykle, M. H., and Cowling, W. R. (1988). Failure to thrive in older persons: A concept derived. *The Gerontologist 28* (6): 809–12.

Briggs, T. (1983). *A Basic Guide for Understanding Guardianship and Conservatorship in Missouri.* Columbia, MO: Missouri Advocacy Services.

Brody, E. (1985). Parent care as a normative family stress. *The Gerontologist 25* (1): 19–29.

Brody, B. A., and Engelhardt, H. T., Jr. (1987). *Bioethics: Readings and Cases.* Englewood Cliffs, NJ: Prentice-Hall.

Brown, L. J., Potter, J. F., and Foster, B. B. (1990). Caregiver burden should be evaluated during geriatric assessment. *Journal of the American Geriatrics Society 38* (4): 455–60.

Brown, S. (1985). *Treating the Alcoholic: A Developmental Model of Recovery.* New York: John Wiley and Sons.

Burda, D. (1987). The nation looks for new ways to finance care for the aged. *Hospitals* (September 20): 48–55.

Burnside, I. (1988). Sleep, rest, and energy. In I. Burnside (ed.), *Nursing and the Aged* (3rd ed.). New York: McGraw-Hill (pp. 213–36).

Butler, R. N., and Lewis, M. I. (1982). *Aging and Mental Health: Positive Psychosocial and Biomedical Approaches* (3rd ed.). St. Louis, MO: C. V. Mosby.

Campbell, L. J., and Cole, K. D. (1987). Geriatric assessment teams. *Clinics in Geriatric Medicine 3*: 99–110.

Canti, T. G., and Korek, J. S. (1987). Prescription of neuroleptics for geriatric nursing home patients. *Hospital and Community Psychiatry 40* (6): 645–47.

Carter, E. A., and McGoldrick, M. (eds.) (1988). *The Changing Family Life Cycle* (2d ed.). New York: Gardner.

Chadwick, R., and Russell, J. (1989). Hospital discharge of frail elderly people: Social and ethical considerations in the discharge decision-making process. *Ageing and Society 9*: 277–95.

Childress, J. F. (1982). *Who Should Decide? Paternalism in Health Care*. New York: Oxford University Press.

Christison, C., Christison, G., and Blazer, D. G. (1989). Late-life schizophrenia and paranoid disorders. In E. W. Busse and D. G. Blazer (eds.), *Geriatric Psychiatry*. Washington, DC: American Psychiatric Press (pp. 403–14).

Clark, A. N. G., Mankikar, G. D., and Gray, I. (1975). Diogenes syndrome: A clinical study of gross neglect in old age. *The Lancet 1* (790): 366–68.

Cohen, C. I., Stastny, P., Perlick, D., and Samuelly, I. (1988). Cognitive deficits among aging schizophrenic patients residing in the community. *Hospital and Community Psychiatry 39*: 557–59.

Cohen, E. S. (1985). Nursing homes and the least-restrictive environment doctrine. In M. B. Kapp, H. E. Pies, Jr., and A. E. Doudera (eds.), *Legal and Ethical Aspects of Health Care for the Elderly*. Ann Arbor: Health Administration Press.

———. (1988). The elder mystique: Constraints on the autonomy of elderly with disabilities. *The Gerontologist 28* (Supplementary Issue): 24–31.

———. (1990). Outcome of schizophrenia into later life: An overview. *The Gerontologist 30* (6): 790–97.

Coleman, N., and Karp, N. (1989). Recent state and federal developments in protective services and elder abuse. *Journal of Elder Abuse and Neglect 1* (2): 51–64.

Collopy, B. J. (1988). Autonomy in long-term care: Some crucial distinctions. *The Gerontologist 28* (Supplementary Issue): 10–17.

Conway, P. (1988). Losses and grief in old age. *Social Casework 69* (9): 541–49.

Conwell, Y., Rotenberg, M. E., and Caine, E. D. (1990). Completed suicide at age 50 and over. *Journal of the American Geriatrics Society 38*: 640–44.

Cornwall, J. A. (1981). Filth, squalor, and lice. *Nursing Mirror 153* (10): 48–49.

Corso, J. F. (1981). *Aging Sensory Systems and Perception*. New York: Praeger (pp. 201–25).

Cotten, P. C., Sison, G. F., and Starr, S. (1981). Comparing elderly mentally retarded and nonretarded individuals: Who are they? What are their needs? *The Gerontologist 21*: 359–65.

Coy, J. A. (1989). Philosophic aspects of patient noncompliance: A critical analysis. *Topics in Geriatric Rehabilitation 4* (3): 52–60.

Culver, C. M. (1985). The clinical determination of competence. In M. B. Kapp, H. E. Pies, Jr., and A. E. Doudera (eds.), *Legal and Ethical Aspects of Health Care for the Elderly*. Ann Arbor: Health Administration Press.

Cybulska, E., and Rucinski, J. (1986). Gross self-neglect in old age. *British Journal of Hospital Medicine 36* (12): 21–25.

Davis-Berman, J. (1990). Physical self-efficacy, perceived physical status, and depressive symptomatology in older adults. *Journal of Psychology 124* (2): 207–15.

Delehanty, M. J. (1985). Health care and inhome environments. In M. P. Janicki and H. M. Wisniewski (eds.), *Aging and Developmental Disabilities: Issues and Approaches*. Baltimore: Paul H. Brookes.

Detweiler, B. (1988). The vexing problem of elder abuse. *Public Welfare 46* (2): 5–6.

DeWeaver, K. L. (1983). Deinstitutionalization of the developmentally disabled. *Social Work 28*: 435–39.

Dilman, V. M. (1981). *The Law of Deviation of Homeostasis and Diseases of Aging*. Boston: John Wright.

Diokno, A. C., Brook, B. M., Brown, M. B., and Herzog, A. R. (1986) Prevalence of urinary incontinence and other urological symptoms in the noninstitutionalized elderly. *Journal of Urology 136*: 1022–25.

Dubin, T. (1987). Profiles of neglect & APS interventions. Presented at the American Public Welfare Association & National Association of State Units on Aging National Conference on Elder Abuse. Washington, DC, January.

Dubler, N. N. (1987). The dependent elderly: Legal rights and responsibilities in agent custody. In S. S. Spicker, S. R. Ingman, and I. R. Lawson (eds.), *Ethical Dimensions of Geriatric Care: Value Conflicts for the 21st Century*. Boston: Reidel.

———. (1988). Improving the discharge planning process: Distinguishing between coercion and choice. *The Gerontologist 28* (Supplementary Issue): 76–81.

Dudley, J. R. (1987). Speaking for themselves: People who are labeled as mentally retarded. *Social Work 32*: 80–82.

Dudovitz, N. S. (1985). The least restrictive alternative. *Generations 10*: 39–41.

Duffy, M. (1984). Aging and the family: Intergenerational psychodynamics. *Psychotherapy 21* (3): 342–46.

———. (1986). Techniques and contexts of multigenerational therapy. *Clinical Gerontologist 5* (3/4): 347–62.

Dworkin, G. (1976). Autonomy and behavior control. *Hastings Center Report 6*: 23–28.

Erckenbrack, N., and Klug, C. (1989). What's missing from elderly aftercare. *The Counselor 7* (2): 16–18.

Eyman, R. K., Grossman, H., Tarjan, G., and Miller, C. (1987). *Life Expectancy and Mental Retardation: A Longitudinal Study in a State Residential Facility*. Washington, DC: American Association on Mental Deficiency.

Farnsworth, M. G. (1989). Evaluation of mental competency. *American Family Physician 39* (6): 182–90.

Favazza, O. R. (1989). Why patients mutilate themselves. *Hospital and Community Psychiatry 40* (2): 137–45.

Fiegener, J. J., Fiegener, M., and Meszaros, J. (1989). Policy implications of a statewide survey of elder abuse. *Journal of Elder Abuse and Neglect 1* (2): 39–58.

Folmar, S., and Wilson, H. (1989). Social behavior and physical restraints. *The Gerontologist 29* (5): 650–53.
Foxx, R. M. (1982). *Increasing Behaviors of Severely Autistic Persons.* Champaign, IL: Research Press.
Fredriksen, K. I. (1989). Adult protective services: Changes with the introduction of mandatory reporting. *Journal of Elder Abuse and Neglect 1* (2): 59–70.
Gadow, S. (1980). Medicine, ethics, and the elderly. *The Gerontologist 20:* 680–85.
Gallo, J. J., Reichel, W., and Andersen, L. (1988). *Handbook of Geriatric Assessment.* Rockville, MD: Aspen.
Gerfo, M. (1980). Three ways of reminiscence in theory and practice. *Journal of Aging and Human Development 12:* 39–48.
Goldfarb, A. I. (1969). The psychodynamics of dependency and the search for aid. In R. A. Kalish (ed.), *Dependencies of Old People.* Occasional Papers in Gerontology. Ann Arbor: Wayne State University Institute of Gerontology (pp. 27–37).
Gomberg, E., and Lisansky, S. (1988). Overview: Issues of alcohol use and abuse in the elderly population. *Pride Institute Journal of Long-Term Home Health Care 7* (2): 4–17.
Goodwin, J. S., Goodwin, J. M., and Garry, P. J. (1983). Association between nutritional status and cognitive functioning in a healthy elderly population. *Journal of the American Medical Association 249:* 2917–21.
Gordis, E. (1988) Alcoholism treatment and older Americans. *Alcohol Alert,* No. 2. Rockville, MD: National Institute on Alcohol Abuse and Alcoholism.
Graham, K. (1986). Identifying and measuring alcohol abuse among the elderly: Serious problems with existing instrumentation. *Journal of Studies on Alcohol 47* (4): 322–25.
Grannum v. Berard, 442 P. 2d 812 (Wash. 1967).
Greene, R. (1986). The functional-age model of intergenerational therapy: A social casework model. *Clinical Gerontologist 5* (3/4): 335–45.
Grossman, H. J. (1983). Definitions. In H. J. Grossman (ed.), *Classification in Mental Retardation.* Washington, DC: American Association on Mental Deficiency.
Gruenberg, E. M. (1967). The social breakdown syndrome: Some origins. *American Journal of Psychiatry 123* (12): 1481–89.
Gruenberg, E. M., Brandon, S., and Kasius, R. V. (1966). Identifying cases of the social breakdown syndrome. *Milbank Memorial Fund Quarterly 44* (January, Part II): 150–55.
Gruenberg, E. M., Snow, H. B., and Bennett, C. L. (1969). Preventing the social breakdown syndrome. In F. C. Redlich (ed.), *Social Psychiatry.* Baltimore: Williams and Wilkins (pp. 179–92).
Gruenberg, E. M., and Zusman, J. (1964). The natural history of schizophrenia. *International Psychiatry Clinics 1* (4): 699–710.
Guccione, A. A. (1988). Compliance and patient autonomy: Ethical and legal limits to professional dominance. *Topics in Geriatric Rehabilitation 3* (3): 62–73.
Gurland, B. J. (1976). The comparative frequency of depression in various adult age groups. *Journal of Gerontology 31:* 283–92.
Haley, J. (1987). *Problem-Solving Therapy* (2d ed.). San Francisco, CA: Jossey-Bass.

Hartman, A., and Laird, J. (1983). *Family Centered Social Work Practice.* New York: Free Press.

Hauber, F., Rolegard, L. L., and Bruininks, R. H. (1985). Characteristics of residential services for older/elderly mentally retarded persons. In M. P. Janicki and H. M. Wisniewski (eds.), *Aging and Developmental Disabilities: Issues and Approaches.* Baltimore: Paul H. Brookes.

Havighurst, R. J. (1951). *Developmental Tasks and Education.* New York: Longmans.

Hawranik, P. (1985). Caring for aging parents: Divided allegiances. *Journal of Gerontological Nursing 11* (10): 19–22.

Helford, M., and Crapo, L. M. (1990). Screening for thyroid disease. *Annals of Internal Medicine 112*: 840–49.

Herst, L. D. (1983). Emergency psychiatry for the elderly. *Psychiatric Clinics of North America 6*: 271–80.

Hickey, T. (1981). *Health and Aging.* Monterey: Brook/Cole.

Hickey, T., Dean, K., and Holstein, B. E. (1986). Emerging trends in gerontology and geriatrics: Implications for the self-care of the elderly. *Social Science and Medicine 23* (12): 1363–69.

High, D. M. (1987). Planning for decisional incapacity: A neglected area in ethics and aging. *Journal of the American Geriatrics Society 35*: 814–20.

Hightower, D., Heckert, A., and Schmidt, W. (1990). Elderly nursing home residents' need for public guardianship in Tennessee. *Journal of Elder Abuse and Neglect 2* (3–4): 105–22.

Himmelfarb, S., and Murrell, S. A. (1984). The prevalence and correlates of anxiety symptoms in older adults. *Journal of Psychology 116*: 159–67.

Hing, E. (1981). *Characteristics of Nursing Home Residents, Health Status, and Care Received.* U.S. DHHS Publication No. (PHS) 81-1712, April.

_____. (1987). *Use of Nursing Homes by the Elderly: Preliminary Data from the 1985 Nursing Home Survey.* U.S. DHHS, NCHS Advance Data No. 135, May 14.

Hoffman, N. G., and Harrison, P. (1989). Characteristics of the older patient in chemical dependency treatment. *The Counselor 7* (2): 11.

Hofland, B. F. (1990). Introduction. *Generations 14* (Supplement): 5–8.

Holman, A. M. (1983). *Family Assessment: Tools for Understanding and Intervention.* Beverly Hills, CA: Sage.

Holstein, B. E. (1986). Health related behavior and aging: Conceptual issues. In K. Dean, T. Hickey, and B. E. Holstein (eds.), *Self-Care and Health in Old Age.* London: Croom-Helm (pp. 35–57).

House, A., and Hodges, J. (1988). Persistent denial of handicap after infarction of the right basal ganglia: A case study. *Journal of Neurology, Neurosurgery, and Psychiatry 51*: 112–15.

Hudson, M. F. (1989). Analysis of the concepts of elder mistreatment: Abuse and neglect. *Journal of Elder Abuse and Neglect 1* (1): 5–25.

Jackson, D. L., and Youngner, S. (1979). Patient autonomy and "death with dignity." *New England Journal of Medicine 301*: 404–8.

Jacobson, J. W., Sutton, M. S., and Janicki, M. P. (1985). Demography and characteristics of aging anda ged mentally retarded persons. In M. P. Janicki and H. M. Wisniewski (eds.), *Aging and Developmental Disabilities: Issues and Approaches.* Baltimore: Paul H. Brookes.

Janicki, M. P. (1986). Older mentally handicapped persons residing at home and in institutions. *British Journal of Mental Subnormality 32*: 30–36.

Janicki, M. P., Ackerman, L., and Jacobson, J. (1985). State developmental disabilities/aging plans and planning for an older developmentally disabled population. *Mental Retardation 23*: 297–301.

Janicki, M. P., Seltzer, M. M., and Krauss, M. W. (1987). *Contemporary Issues in the Aging of Persons with Mental Retardation and Other Developmental Disabilties*. Washington, DC: National Rehabilitation Center.

Johnson Institute Books (1987). *How to Use Intervention in Your Professional Practice*. Minneapolis: Johnson Institute Books.

Kahana, E. F., and Kiyak, A. H. (1984). Attitudes and behavior of staff in facilities for the aged. *Research on Aging 6* (3): 395–416.

Kane, R. A. (1990). Assessing the elderly client. In A. Monk (ed.), *Handbook of Gerontological Services* (2d ed.). New York: Columbia University Press (pp. 55–89).

Kane, R. A., and Kane, R. L. (1981). *Assessing the Elderly: A Practical Guide to Measurement*. Lexington, MA: Lexington Books.

———. (1986). Self-care and health care: Inseparable but equal for the well-being of the old. In K. Dean, T. Hickey, and B. E. Holstein (eds.), *Self-Care and Health in Old Age*. London: Croom-Helm (pp. 251–83).

Kapp, M. B. (1985). Adult protective services: Convincing the patient to consent. In M. B. Kapp, H. E. Pies, Jr., and A. E. Doudera (eds.), *Legal and Ethical Aspects of Health Care for the Elderly*. Ann Arbor: Health Administration Press.

———. (1988). Forcing services on at-risk older adults: When doing good is not so good. *Social Work in Health Care 13* (4): 1–13.

———. (1990). Evaluating decision-making capacity in the elderly: A review of recent literature. *Journal of Elder Abuse and Neglect 2* (3–4): 15–29.

Kapp, M. B., and Bigot, A. (1985). *Geriatrics and the Law: Patient Rights and Professional Responsibilities*. New York: Springer.

Kasl, S. V., Ostfeld, A. M., Brody, G. M., Snell, L., and Price, C. A. (1980). Effects of "involuntary" relocation on the health and behavior of the elderly. In S. G. Haynes and M. Feinlieb (eds.), *Epidemiology of Aging*. U.S. DHHS, NIH Publication No. 80-969, July.

Kastenbaum, R., and Mishara, B. (1971). Premature death and self-injurious behavior in old age. *Geriatrics 26*: 70–81.

Kemp, B. J. (1988). Motivation, rehabilitation, and aging: A conceptual model. *Topics in Geriatric Rehabilitation 3* (3): 41–51.

Kerr, M. E., and Bowen, M. (1988). *Family Evaluation*. New York: Norton.

Kofoed, A. A., Polson, R. L., Atkinson, R. M., Toth, R. L., and Turner, J. A. (1987). Treatment compliance of older alcoholics: An elder-specific approach is superior to "mainstreaming." *Journal of Studies on Alcohol 48* (1): 47–51.

Kohrs, M. B., Wang, L. L., Eklund, D., Paulsen, B., and O'Neal, R. (1979). The association of obesity with socioeconomic factors in Missouri. *American Journal of Clinical Nutrition 32*: 2120–28.

Kola, L. A., Kosberg, J. I., and Wegner-Burch, K. (1980). Perceptions of the treatment responsibilities for the alcoholic elderly client. *Social Work in Health Care 6* (2): 69–76.

Kolevzon, M. S., and Green, R. G. (1985). *Family Therapy Models.* New York: Springer.
Klosterkotter, J., and Peters, U. H. (1985). Das diogenes-syndrome. *Fortschr. Neurol. Psychiat. 53* (1): 427–34.
Kuyper, J. A., and Bengtson, V. L. (1973). Social breakdown and competence: A model of normal aging. *Human Development 16* (3): 182–201.
Lakin, K. C. (1985). Service systems and settings for mentally retarded people. In K. C. Lakin, B. Hill, and R. H. Bruininks (eds.), *An Analysis of Medicaid's Intermediate Care Facility for the Mentally Retarded (ICF/MR) Program.* Minneapolis: University of Minnesota, Department of Educational Psychology.
Lazarus, R. S., and Folkman, S. (1984). *Stress, Appraisal, and Coping.* New York: Springer.
Levin, L. S., Katz, A. H., and Holst, E. (1976). *Self-Care: Lay Initiatives in Health.* New York: Prodist.
Liang, J., and Jow-Ching Fu, E. (1986). Estimating lifetime risks of nursing home residents: A further note. *The Gerontologist 26* (5): 560–63.
Lieberman, M. A., and Tobin, S. S. (1983). *The Experience of Old Age: Stress, Coping, and Survival.* New York: Basic Books.
Lipowski, Z. J. (1989). Delirium and the elderly patient. *New England Journal of Medicine 320*: 578–82.
Lott, I. T., and Lai, F. (1982). Dementia in Down's syndrome: Observations from a neurology clinic. *Applied Research in Mental Retardation 3*: 233–39.
Mace, N. L., and Rabins, P. V. (1981). *The 36-Hour Day.* Baltimore: Johns Hopkins University Press.
MacLeod, A. D. (1988). Self-neglect of spinal injured patients. *Paraplegia 26*: 340–49.
Macmillan, D., and Shaw, P. (1966). Senile breakdown in standards of personal and environmental cleanliness. *British Medical Journal 2* (5521): 1032–37.
Magni, G., and De Leo, D. (1984). Anxiety and depression in geriatric and adult medical inpatients: A comparison. *Psychological Reports 55*: 607–12.
Mark, V. W., and Heilman, K. M. (1990). Bodily neglect and orientational biases in unilateral neglect syndrome and normal subjects. *Neurology 40*: 640–43.
Markson, E., Kwoh, A., and Cumming, J. (1971). Alternatives to hospitalization for psychiatrically ill geriatric patients. *American Journal of Psychiatry 27*: 1055–62.
Martin, G., and Pear, J. (1988). *What It Is and How To Do It* (3rd ed.). Englewood Cliffs, NJ: Prentice-Hall.
Marton, K. I., Sox, H. C., and Krupp, J. R. (1981). Involuntary weight loss: Diagnostic and prognostic significance. *Annals of Internal Medicine 95*: 568–74.
Maslow, A. H. (1954). *Motivation and Personality.* New York: Harper and Row.
McConnel, C. (1984). A note on the lifetime risk of nursing home residency. *The Gerontologist 24* (2): 193–98.
McIntosh, J. L., and Hubbard, R. W. (1988). Indirect self-destructive behavior among the elderly: A review with case examples. *Journal of Gerontological Social Work 13* (1-a): 37–48.
McKay, J. B. (1984). Protective services give elders more autonomy. *Generations 8* (3): 10–13.

McNiel, D. E., and Binder, R. L. (1987). Predictive value of judgments of dangerousness in emergency civil commitment. *American Journal of Psychiatry 144*: 197–200.
Mechanic, D. (1960). Illness behavior and medical diagnosis. *Journal of Health and Social Behavior 1*: 86–94.
———. (1968). *Medical Sociology: A Selective View*. New York: The Free Press.
Meisel, A., Roth, C. H., and Lidz, C. W. (1977). Toward a model of the legal doctrine of informed consent. *American Journal of Psychiatry 134*: 285–89.
Mercer, S. O., and Kane, R. A. (1979). Helplessness and hopelessness in the institutionalized aged: A field experiment. *Health and Social Work 4* (1): 91–116.
Metzger, L. (1988). *From Denial to Recovery: Counseling Problem Drinkers, Alcoholics, and Their Families*. San Francisco: Jossey-Bass.
Meyers, B. S., Kalayam, B., and Mei-Tal, V. (1984). Late-onset delusional depression: A distinct clinical entity? *Journal of Clinical Psychiatry 45*: 347–49.
Mill, J. S. (1863). *On Liberty*. Boston: Ticknor and Fields.
Miller, D. A. (1981). The sandwich generation: Adult children of the aging. *Social Work 26*: 419–23.
Miniszek, N. A. (1983). Development of Alzheimer's disease in Down's syndrome individuals. *American Journal of Mental Deficiency 87*: 377–85.
Minuchin, S. (1974). *Families and Family Therapy*. Cambridge, MA: Harvard University Press.
Mirotznik, J., and Ruskin, A. (1984). Interinstitutional relocation and its effect on health. *The Gerontologist 24* (3): 286–91.
Mishara, B. L., and Kastenbaum, R. (1973). Self-injurious behavior and environmental change in the institutionalized elderly. *International Journal of Aging and Human Development 4* (2): 133–45.
Mishara, B. L., Robertson, B., and Kastenbaum, R. (1973). Self-injurious behavior in the elderly. *The Gerontologist 13* (3): 311–14.
Morewitz, J. H. (1988). Evaluation of excessive daytime sleepiness in the elderly. *Journal of the American Geriatrics Society 36*: 324–30.
Morley, J. E. (1986). Nutritional status of the elderly. *American Journal of Medicine 81*: 679–95.
Morris, C. H., Hope, R. A., and Fairburn, C. G. (1989). Eating habits in dementia: A descriptive study. *British Journal of Psychiatry 154*: 801–6.
Moskop, J. C. (1987). The moral limits to federal funding for kidney disease. *Hastings Center Report 17*: 11–15.
Mowry, B. J., and Burvill, P. W. (1990). Screening the elderly in the community for psychiatric disorder. *Australian and New Zealand Journal of Psychiatry 24* (2): 203–6.
National Association of Adult Protective Services Administrators (1990, October). *Position Paper on Self-Neglect* (Available from Marilyn Whalen, TDHS, 400 Deaderick St., Nashville, TN 37249-97003).
National Association of Social Workers (1982). Changes in NASW family policy. *NASW News 27* (2): 10.
National Association of State Units on Aging and American Public Welfare Association (1988). *Adult Protective Services: Programs in State Social*

Service Agencies and State Units on Aging. Washington, DC: American Public Welfare Association.

Noelker, L. S., and Bass, D. M. (1989). Home care for elderly persons: Linkage between formal and informal caregivers. *Journal of Gerontology 44* (2): 563–70.

Office of Technology Assessment (1987). *Life-Sustaining Technologies and the Elderly.* Washington, DC: U.S. Government Printing Office.

O'Rawe, A. M. (1982). Nursing care study: Self-neglect — a challenge for nursing. *Nursing Times 78* (46): 1932–36.

Orem, D. (1980). *Nursing Concepts of Practice* (1st ed.). New York: McGraw-Hill.

———. (1985). *Nursing: Concepts of Practice* (2d ed.). New York: McGraw-Hill.

Orrel, M. W., Sahabian, B. J., and Bergmann, K. (1989). Self-neglect and frontal lobe dysfunction. *British Journal of Psychiatry 155*: 101–5.

Palmore, E. (1976). Total change of institutionalization among the aged. *The Gerontologist 16* (6): 504–7.

Parsons, R. J., and Cox, E. O. (1989). Family mediation in elder caregiving decisions: An empowerment intervention. *Social Work 34* (2): 122–26.

Perez, V. S. (1989). Dual diagnosis in the older adult: Diagnosis and treatment issues. *The Counselor 7* (2): 12–14.

Pinkston, E. M., and Linsk, N. L. (1984). *Care of the Elderly: A Family Approach.* New York: Pergamon Press.

Potter, J. F., and Jameton, A. (1986). Respecting the choices of neglected elders: Autonomy or abuse. In M. W. Galibraith (ed.), *Elder Abuse: Perspectives on an Emerging Crisis.* Kansas City: Mid-America Congress on Aging (Vol. 3, pp. 95–109).

Poulshock, S. W., and Deimling, G. T. (1984). Families caring for elders in residence: Issues in the measurement of burden. *Journal of Gerontology 39* (2): 230–39.

President's Commission for the Study of Ethical Problems in Medicine and Biomedical and Behavioral Research (1982). *Making Health Care Decisions: The Ethical and Legal Implications of Informed Consent in the Patient-Practitioner Relationship.* Washington, DC: U.S. Government Printing Office.

Quinn, M. J. (1985). Elder abuse and neglect raise new dilemmas. *Generations 10*: 22–25.

Quinn, M. J., and Tomita, S. K. (1986). *Elder Abuse and Neglect: Causes, Diagnosis, and Intervention Strategies.* New York: Springer.

Radebaugh, T. S., Hooper, F. J., and Gruenberg, E. M. (1987). The social breakdown syndrome in the elderly population living in the community: The helping study. *British Journal of Psychiatry 151*: 341–46.

Ramsdell, J. W., Sward, J. A., Jackson, J. E., and Renvall, M. (1989). The yield of a home visit in the assessment of geriatric patients. *Journal of the American Geriatrics Society 37*: 14–17.

Ramsden, E. L. (1988). Compliance and motivation. *Topics in Geriatric Rehabilitation 3* (3): 1–14.

Rathbone-McCuan, E. (1991). Family counseling: An emerging approach in clinical gerontology. In P. Kim (ed.), *Serving the Elderly: Skills for Practice.* Hawthorne, NY: Aldine de Gruyter (pp. 51–66).

———. (in press). Aged adult protective service clients: People of unrecognized potential. In M. D. Saleebey (ed.), *Power in the People: The Strengths Perspective in Social Work Practice*. White Plains: Longmans.
Rathbone-McCuan, E., and Bricker-Jenkins, M. (1988). *Self-Neglect and Adult Protective Services*. Tennessee Department of Human Services.
Rathbone-McCuan, E., and Hashimi, J. (1982). *Isolated Elders*. Rockville, MD: Aspen.
Reagan, J. T. (1986). Management of nurses' aides in long-term care settings. *The Journal of Long-Term Care Administration* (Summer): 9–14.
Reed, P. G., and Leonard, V. E. (1989). An analysis of the concept of self-neglect. *Advances in Nursing Science 12* (1): 39–53.
Reese, H. W., and Rodeheaver, D. (1985). Problem solving and complex decision making. In J. E. Birren and K. W. Schaie (eds.), *Handbook of the Psychology of Aging* (2d ed.). New York: Van Nostrand Reinhold (pp. 474–99).
Reichel, J. (1989). Pulmonary problems in the elderly. In W. Reichel (ed.), *Clinical Aspects of Aging* (3rd ed.). Baltimore: Williams & Wilkins.
Reifler, B. V., and Eisdorfer, C. (1980). A clinic for the impaired elderly and their families. *American Journal of Psychiatry 137*: 1399–1403.
Richards, B. W. (1976). Health and longevity. In J. Wortis (ed.), *Mental Retardation and Developmental Disabilities: An Annual Review*. Vol. 8. New York: Brunner-Mazel.
Robertson, A. (1989). Treatment issue of the older adult. *The Counselor 7* (2): 8–10.
Robinson, B. C. (1983). Validation of a caregiver strain index. *Journal of Gerontology 38*: 344–48.
Robinson, R. G., Kubos, K. L., Starr, L. B., Rao, K., and Price, T. R. (1984). The mood disorders in stroke patients: Importance of location of lesion. *Brain 107*: 81–93.
Rodin, J. (1986). Aging and health: Effects of the sense of control. *Science*: 1271–76.
Roe, P. F. (1977). Self-neglect. *Age and Ageing 6* (3): 192–94.
———. (1987). A letter. *British Journal of Hospital Medicine 37* (1): 83–84.
Rolland, J. S. (1987). Chronic illness and the life cycle: A conceptual framework. *Family Process 26*: 204–21.
Rose, B. D. (1989). Hypo-osmolal states-hyponatremia. In *Clinical Physiology of Acid-Base and Electrolyte Disorders* (3rd ed.). New York: McGraw-Hill.
Rose, T., and Janicki, M. P. (1986). Older mentally retarded adults: A forgotten population. *Aging Network News 3*: 17–19.
Rosendahl, P., and Ross, V. (1982). Does your behavior affect your patient's response? *Journal of Gerontological Nursing 8* (10): 572–75.
Rothbaum, F., Weisz, J., and Snyder, S. (1982). Changing the world and changing the self: A two-process model of perceived control. *Journal of Personality and Social Psychology 42*: 5–37.
Rounds, L. R. (1985). A study of selected environmental variables associated with noninstitutional settings where there is abuse or neglect of the elderly. *Dissertation Abstracts International 45* (7): 2221-A.
Rovner, B. W., Kafonek, S., Filipp, L., Lucas, M. J., and Folstein, M. F. (1986). Prevalence of mental illness in a community nursing home. *American Journal of Psychiatry 143*: 1449.
Rowles, G. D., and Reinharz, S. (1988). Qualitative gerontology: Themes and

challenges. In S. Rinharz and G. D. Rowles (eds.), *Qualitative Gerontology*. New York: Springer.

Rubenstine, L. V., Calkins, D. R., Greenfield, S., Jette, A. M., Meenarr, R. F., Nevins, M. A., Rubenstein, L. Z., Wasson, J. H., and Williams, M. E. (1989). Health status assessment for elderly patients: Report of the society of general internal medicine task force on health assessment. *Journal of the American Geriatrics Society 37* (6): 562–69.

Rubenstein, L. Z. (1987). Geriatric assessment: An overview of its impacts. *Clinics in Geriatric Medicine 3*: 1–15.

Rubin, E. H. (1988). Aging and mania. *Psychiatric Developments 6*: 329–37.

Salend, E., Kane, R. A., Satz, M., and Pynoos, J. (1984). Elder abuse reporting: Limitations of status. *The Gerontologist 24* (1): 61–67.

Sandstead, H. H. (1985). Some thoughts on nutrition and aging. *Drug-Nutrient Interactions 4*: 83–85.

Satir, V. (1988). *The New Peoplemaking*. Mountain View, CA: Science & Behavior Books.

Schene, P., and Ward, S. F. (1988). The relevance of child protection experience. *Public Welfare 46* (2): 14–21.

Schmidt, W. C. (1985). Guardianship: Public and private. In M. B. Kapp, H. E. Pies, Jr., and A. W. Doudera (eds.), *Legal and Ethical Aspects of Health Care for the Elderly*. Ann Arbor: Health Administration Press.

J. B. Schneewind, ed. (1983). *An Enquiry Concerning the Principles of Morals*. Indianapolis: Hackett.

Select Committee on Aging (1985). *America's Elderly at Risk*. Committee Publication No. 99-508. Washington, DC: U.S. Government Printing Office.

Seltzer, M. M., and Krauss, M. W. (1987). *Aging and Mental Retardation: Extending the Continuum*. Washington, DC: American Association on Mental Deficiency.

Seltzer, M. M., Krauss, M. W., Litchfield, L. C., and Modlish, N. J. (1989). Utilization of aging network services by elderly persons with mental retardation. *The Gerontologist 29*: 234–38.

Serkin, E. (1987). Elderly alcoholics and their adult children. *Focus* (September–October): 12–13, 23–25.

Shaughnessy, P. W. (1989). Quality of nursing home care. *Generations 13* (1): 17–20.

Sheikh, J. I., and Yesavage, J. A. (1986). Geriatric Depression Scale (GDS): Recent evidence and development of a shorter version. In T. L. Brink (ed.), *Clinical Gerontology*. New York: Haworth Press.

Sider, R. C., and Clements, C. D. (1984). Patients' ethical obligation for their health. *Journal of Medical Ethics 10*: 138–42.

Simon, R. (1989). Silent suicide in the elderly. *Bulletin of the American Academy of Psychiatry and the Law 17*: 83–95.

Smith, D. A. (1990). New rules for prescribing psychotherapies in nursing homes. *Geriatrics 45*: 44–56.

Solomon, K. (1990). Learned helplessness in the elderly: Theoretical and clinical implications. *Occupational Therapy in Mental Health 10*: 31–51.

Stanley, B., Stanley, M., Guido, J., and Garvin, L. (1988). The functional competency of elderly at risk. *The Gerontologist 28* (Supplementary Issue): 53–58.

Strahan, G. (1987). *Nursing Home Characteristics: Preliminary Data from the 1985 National Nursing Home Survey*. Advance data No. 131, March 27.
Tarjan, G., Wright, S. W., Eyman, R. K., and Keeran, C. V. (1973). Natural history of mental retardation: Some aspects of epidemiology. *American Journal of Mental Deficiency 77*: 369–79.
Tennessee Department of Human Services (1986, July). *Protective Services for Adults*. Nashville, TN: Commissioner of Human Services (Ch. 16, pp. 1–78).
Thomas, D. R. (1989). Differential diagnosis of dementing diseases. *Journal of Mississippi State Medical Association 30* (12): 391–94.
Thomasma, D. C. (1984). Freedom, dependency, and the care of the very old. *Journal of the American Geriatrics Society 32* (12): 906–14.
Tobias, C. R., Lippman, S., Tully, E., Pary, R., and Tarns, D. M. (1989). Delirium in the elderly. *Postgraduate Medicine 85*: 117–30.
Townsend, A. L., and Poulshock, S. W. (1986). Intergenerational perspectives on impaired elder support network. *Journal of Gerontology 41* (1): 101–9.
U.S. General Accounting Office (1986). *An Aging Society: Meeting the Needs of the Elderly while Responding to Rising Federal Costs*. GAO-HRD-86-135. Washington, DC: U.S. Government Printing Office.
U.S. Senate, Special Committee on Aging (1989). *Aging America: Trends and Projections*. Washington, DC: U.S. Government Printing Office.
U.S. Senate, Special Committee on Aging, Subcommittee on Long-Term Care: Supporting Paper No. 7 (1976). *The Role of Nursing Homes in Caring for Discharged Mental Patients (and the Birth of a For-Profit Boarding Home Industry)*. Washington, DC: U.S. Government Printing Office.
Van der Kolk, B. A. (1987). *Psychological Trauma*. Washington, DC: American Psychiatric Press.
Vandeputte, C. (1989). Special detox needs of the elderly. *The Counselor 7* (2): 19–20.
Vickers, R. (1976). The therapeutic milieu and the older depressed patient. *Journal of Gerontology 31*: 314–17.
———. (1988). Medical aspects of aging. In L. W. Lazarus (ed.), *Essentials of Geriatric Psychiatry*. New York: Springer (pp. 65–101).
Walsh, F. (1982). *Normal Family Processes*. New York: Guilford.
———. (1988). The family in later life. In E. A. Carter and M. McGoldrick (eds.), *The Family Life Cycle* (2d ed.). New York: Gardner (pp. 311–32).
Walz, T., Harper, D., and Wilson, J. (1986). The aging developmentally disabled person: A review. *The Gerontologist 26*: 622–29.
Wetle, T. (1985). Long-term care: A taxonomy of issues. *Generations 10*: 30–34.
Williams, M. (1984). Alcohol and the elderly: An overview. *Alcohol Health and Research World* (Spring): 4–51
Williamson, Donald S. (1981). Termination of the intergenerational hierarchical boundary between the first and second generations: A new stage in the family. *Journal of Marital and Family Therapy 7* (4): 441–51.
Wisniewski, H. M., and Marz, G. S. (1985). Aging, Alzheimer's disease, and developmental disabilities. In M. P. Janicki and H. M. Wisniewski (eds.), *Aging and Developmental Disabilities: Issues and Approaches*. Baltimore: Paul H. Brookes.
Wolf, R. S. (1988). The evolution of policy: A 10-year retrospective. *Public Welfare 46* (2): 7–13.

Woodruff, J. C., Denman, H., and Halpin, G. (1988). Changing elderly persons' attitudes toward mental health professionals. *The Gerontologist 28*: 800–2.

Woods, N. (1989). Conceptualization of self-care: Toward health-oriented models. *Advances in Nursing Science 12* (1): 1–13.

Woolfson, P. (1988). Cross-cultural families: The Franco-Americans. In E. Rathbone-McCuan and B. Havens (eds.), *North American Elders: United States and Canadian Perspectives*. Westport, CT: Greenwood Press (pp. 271–80).

Zarit, S. H., Eiler, J., and Hassinger, M. (1985). Clinical assessment. In J. E. Birren and K. W. Schaie (eds.), *Handbook of the Psychology of Aging* (2d ed.). New York: Van Nostrand Reinhold (pp. 747–54).

Zellman, H. E. (1978). Unusual aspects of myxedema. *Geriatrics 23*: 140–48.

Zola, I. F. (1986). Reasons for noncompliance and failure of the elderly to seek care. In R. Moskowitz and M. R. Haugh (eds.), *Arthritis and the Elderly*. New York: Springer (pp. 72–84).

Zuckerman, C. (1987a). Conclusions and guidelines for practice. *Generations 11*: 67–73.

―――. (1987b). An attorney's view. *Generations* (Summer): 60–61.

Zusman, J. (1967). Some explanations of the changing appearance of psychotic patients. *International Journal of Psychiatry 3* (4): 216–37.

Index

abuse. *See* elder abuse
acting-out behavior, 52
activities of daily living (ADL), 47
adaptive compensation, for self-care, 16–20
Addison's disease, 58
adjustment disorder of late life, 47
Administration on Aging, U.S., 145, 147
adult protective services (APS), 159–60; and consciousness raising about neglect/abuse issues, 145–46; and coordination of multiscore services by staff, 158–59; definition of, 144; elder self-neglect issues in Tennessee, 152–59; national perspective on protection and self-neglect, 147–48; practice philosophy of, 153–54; and self-neglect, 148–52, 171
advocate, professional role of, 23–24, 31, 146
aftercare, 141
aging, in developmentally disabled, 108–11
AIDS, 50, 56, 58, 61
Albany model of assessment, 68–70
alcoholism, 51; definition of alcohol problem, 128; intervention during on-going abuse, 140–42; and liver failure, 61; and malnutrition, 60, 61; onset of, 129, 142; and self-neglect, 10, 12, 14; symptoms of, 51. *See also* elder alcoholic self-neglect
Alzheimer's disease, 8, 42, 49, 69, 110; and dementia, 50; and feeding problems, 60
American Association of Retired Persons, 109
American Public Welfare Association, 147
anabolism, effect of disturbances in, 56, 58
anemia, 56
anorexia, 59–60, 61
antacids, and malnutrition, 61
antisocial personality, 51–52
anxiety, 48; characteristics of, 47–48
apathetic hyperthyroidism, 58
apnea, 56
aspiration of food/liquids, 60
assessment: behavioral, 120–21, 165; client resistance to, 66–68; and client vulnerability, 15; court-ordered, 67, 156–57; of decision-making capacity, 151–52; definition of, 164–65; of

developmentally disabled adults, 114, 117–21; family focused, 19, 64–65, 72, 75, 76–79, 165; focus of, 23; for geriatric services, 150–52; goal of, 22–23; of living situation, 117–18; medical, 57–58; mental health, 46–54, 65; multidisciplinary team approach to, 64, 65, 68–70; psychosocial risk, 129–32; recordkeeping for, 66; refinements in, 164–67; of self-care capacity, 166; for self-neglect problems, 63–66; and sex role stereotyping, 65–66; techniques applicable to adult protective services programs, 150–52. *See also* intervention strategies; referrals

assistance: acceptance of and adaptive compensation, 18; refusal of, 7, 14, 34–35, 38–39, 41

Association of Adult Protective Services Administrators (NAAPSA), 146

asthma, 56

atropine analogs, 56

autism, 109

autonomy, 86; application of, 29–30; and informed consent, 30; legal and ethical issues of, for patient, 11, 28–30, 40–41; in nursing home, 95; physical, 167–68; psychological dimension of, 168; spiritual dimension of, 168; tensions between paternalism and, 31

awareness of capacity, 17

awareness of potential, 17

basic needs, concept of, 54–55

behavior: acting-out, 52; assessment of, and self-care skills training, 165; biomedical conditions affecting, 54–58; life-threatening, 95; measuring duration of, 120; measuring form of, 120; measuring frequency of, 120; measuring intensity of, 120–21; measuring latency of, 120

behavioral goals, for older developmentally disabled adults, 117, 118–21

behavior therapy for developmentally disabled adults, 108, 116; assessing living situation, 117–18; case studies, 121–25; goal setting and evaluating existing skills, 118–21

beneficence, 43; application of, 31–32; and cost-benefit assessments, 31–32; and paternalism, 31–32; principle of, 30–31

biomedical considerations, in self-neglect, 46–70

bipolar affective disorders, 54

boarding homes, 91, 115. *See also* institutionalization; nursing home

borderline personality, 52

brain trauma, 50

breathing difficulties, 56

bronchitis, 56, 60

cancer, 60

capacity: assessment of decision-making, 151–52; assessment of self-care, 166; distinction between sanity and, 157

capacity to consent, of elder client, 156–57

Capital District Psychiatric Center's Mobile Geriatric Screening Team (Albany, New York), 68–70

caregiver: psychosocial characteristics of, 64; self-neglect in, 34–35; training for, 28

caregiving system, case study of overwhelmed, 83–84

case identification, 169–70

catabolic wasting, 61

catabolism, effect of disturbances in, 55, 58, 61

cataracts, 57

cerebral palsy, 109

chronic bronchitis, 56

chronic disease, 29, 60, 61, 130–31

Chronic Obstructive Lung Disease (COPD), 56

cleanliness, 7, 10. *See also* personal hygiene

clients: being an advocate for, 23–24, 31; relationship with practitioner, 22;

resistance to assessment, 66–68
clinical directions. *See* research
codependency, 132
commitment, involuntary, 65, 67
communication: distortion of, 57–58; and deafness, 60; in family, 72, 78
community, costs of self-neglect for, 35–37; developmentally disabled adults in, 115–16
compensatory daytime somnolence, 56
competency: and alcoholism, 139–40; and commitment, 67–68; definition of, 29; and ethics of intervention, 39–42; mental, 29–30, 37–38. *See also* assessment
compliance, medical, 10, 98–99, 111, 112; and self-neglect, 9–11
consent: capacity of elder client in, 156–57; informed, 28, 30
conservatorships, 43, 66; and elder alcoholic self-neglect, 139–40
coronary heart disease, 60
cost-benefit assessments, 31–32
court-ordered examination, 67, 156–57
covetousness, 65
crisis intervention, 23
custodianship, 66

dangerous situations, intervention in, 138–39
deafness, 60
decision making, 22, 151, 153; group, in nursing home, 103
defense mechanisms, 47
delegation of responsibility, 19–20
delirium, 49, 69; characteristics of, 50; diagnosis of, 50; differentiation from dementia, 50; symptoms of, 50
dementia, 29, 69; and autonomy, 167; characteristics of, 49; definition of, 97; diagnosis of, 50; differentiation from delirium, 50; and feeding problems, 60
depression, 18, 48, 60; characteristics of, 47–48; diagnosis of, in elderly, 48–49; self-neglect in, 3; treatment of, 42
Developmental Disabilities Act (1984), 108
developmental disability, definition of, 108–9
developmentally disabled adults, 107, 125–26; aging among, 108–11; behavior therapy for, 116–21; case studies of behavior therapy for, 121–25; causes for self-neglecting behavior in, 113–14; physical location and self-neglecting behavior, 115–16; self-neglect issues, 111–12
diabetes, 58, 61, 151
diagnosis. *See* assessment; intervention strategies; referrals
Diagnostic and Statistical Manual of American Psychiatric Association, 47–48, 97
diarrhea, 61
Digoxin, 61
Diogenes syndrome, 5, 128, 168
distributive justice, principle of, 33
Down's syndrome, 110
durable power of attorney, 44
dysfunctional family, case study of, 81–83
dysphagia, 60

early-onset alcoholic, 129
eco-map, 78–79
elder abuse: consciousness raising about, 145–46; national policy on, 145–46; research on, 4
elder alcoholic self-neglect, 127; case studies, 133–36; and chronic health problems, 130–31; definition of, 128–29; and familial role changes, 132; future program development, 143; interrelationship of risk factors, 132; intervention strategies for, 136–42; and isolation, 130; and loss/grief, 130; on-going treatment during recovery, 141–42; psychosocial risk assessment, 129–32; and retirement, 131–32; and social status, 131; treatment potential, 137. *See also* alcoholism
elder protection movement, 144
elder self-neglect: context of, 13–15; in

developmentally disabled adults, 111–21; emerging definition of, 148–50; family focused assessment of, 75; intervention approaches appropriate for, 150–52; major factors in, 15–16; in nursing home, 93–97; and practitioner-client relationship, 22; profile of, 151; research issues, 152–59; resistance to help, 7, 14, 34–35, 38–39, 41; stereotyping of, 4–6, 12, 128. See also self-neglect
electrolyte disturbances, 50
emergency court orders, 157
emphysema, 56
employment issues, and developmentally disabled adults, 112
endangerment, 151
environmental factors, in self-neglecting behavior, 6, 21, 114
epilepsy, 53, 109
ethical issues, 27–28; autonomy, 11, 28–30, 39, 40–41; beneficence, 30–32; case studies, 34–45; community costs of self-neglect, 35–37; and intervention strategies, 9, 39–44, 129; justice, 32–34; personal preferences versus professional judgment, 37–38; right of self-determination, 38–39; self-neglect in caregiver, 34–35
evaluation. See assessment; intervention strategies; referrals
excretion, 58
exercise, 57

family: and assessment, 19, 64, 72, 75, 76–79, 165; and coordination of services, 158–59; communicating with out-of-town, 138; contact with, during institutionalization, 101–2; definition of, 72; developmental tasks of aging, 73; and elder alcoholic, 132; and older developmentally disabled adult, 115–16
family assessment tools: eco-map, 78–79; family mapping, 79; genogram, 79
family systems, 71–74, 88; case illustrations, 79–87; clinical application, 72; components of assessment process, 76–78; family assessment tools, 78–79; family focused assessment of elder self-neglect, 75
financial resources/ability, and self-neglecting behavior, 113
fluids, refusal of, 38–39; and water deprivation, 62–63
food, for nursing home resident, 101–2, 103; refusal of, 38–39, 59–61. See also nutrition
foster homes, 115

generational boundaries, 73
Geriatric Depression Scale, 49
geropsychiatric services, referrals for, 48
glaucoma, 57, 151
Great Britain, eligibility for end-stage renal dialysis in, 32
group decision making, in nursing home, 103
group homes, 91, 115
guardian ad litem, 158
guardianships, 43, 157–58; and elder alcoholic self-neglect, 136, 139–40

health issues, and developmentally disabled adults, 112
health personnel, and noncompliance, 10–11
health status: and elder alcoholic self-neglect, 130–31; and self-neglecting behavior, 114
hearing impairments, 57–58, 60
heart failure, 29, 60
helplessness, 8
helplessness-hopelessness syndrome, 48
hemicorporeal neglect syndrome, 53
histrionic personality, 51–52
homelessness: and developmentally disabled adults, 116; and mental disorders, 51, 53; and network of support in, 74; and self-neglect, 7
hope, loss of, 59–60

hospitalization: involuntary, 43; voluntary, 67
household goods, disposal of, 100
House Select Committee on Aging, Subcommittee on Health and Long-Term Care, 145
housing, for developmentally disabled adults, 112, 115–16
hypochondriacal personality, 52
hyponatremia, 62
hypothermia, 51
hypoxia, 56

impotency, 60
incontinence, 58, 62–63
independence, elders' desire for, 17, 18, 20, 40; and translocation shock, 95–96
informal care, 171–72
informed consent, and autonomy, 28, 30
institutional care settings. *See* nursing home
institutionalization: contact with family during, 101–2; misinformation on, 64–65; self-care in, 91. *See also* nursing homes
instrumental activities of daily living (IADL), 47
intellectual capacity, 29
intergenerational issues: and caregiver-care receiver relationship, 73; and codependency, 132; family history and assessment process, 77
intermittent alcoholic, 129
intervention strategies: and autonomy, 167–68; and coordination of multisource services in, 158–59; in dangerous situations, 138–39; for developmentally disabled adults, 116–21, 121–25; for elder alcoholic self-neglect, 8–9, 14–15, 136–42; for elder self-neglect, 150–52; ethical considerations for, 9, 39–44, 129; legal aspects of, 156–58; during on-going alcohol abuse, 140–41; social, 154–56. *See also* adult protective services (APS); assessment; referrals
involuntary hospitalization, 43

isolation: and elder alcoholic self-neglect, 130–31; in elderly, 74, 79–81

Journal of Elder Abuse and Neglect, 146
justice: allocation of scarce resources, 32; application of, 32–34; distributive, 33; principle of, 32

knowledge building: case identification as source of, 169–70; qualitative studies for, 170–71

late-onset alcoholic, 129
laxatives, and malnutrition, 61
least restrictive alternative, principle of, 44
legal issues. *See* ethical issues
life-threatening behavior, 95
limited guardianship, 157
lithium, 54
liver failure, 61
loss: and elder alcoholic self-neglect, 130; and sense of self, 16; and sense of will, 17
low blood potassium, 62
low-salt syndrome, 62

malnutrition, 7, 51; and alcoholism, 61; protein-calorie, 61–63. *See also* nutrition
manic-depressive reactions, 54
Mann, Marty, 128
meal planning, in nursing home, 103. *See also* nutrition
Medicaid, 92, 151
medical compliance, 10, 98–99; in developmentally disabled adults, 111, 112
medical sociology, 163
Medicare, 59, 92, 109
medication use: and alcoholism, 131–32; compliance, 10; in nursing home, 93; and malnutrition, 61; by psychiatric patient, 10
memory impairment, in alcoholism, 128. *See also* Alzheimer's disease
mental disorders: assessment of, 46–47, 65; and medical compliance, 10; and

protective services, 9; and self-neglect, 8, 12, 13, 46–54; and social breakdown syndrome, 5–6
mental hospitals, 91
mentally retarded population: definition of old age for, 110; estimating size of elderly, 110–11
mental retardation: and life expectation, 54; mild, 109; moderate, 109
mineral disturbance, 62
Mobile Geriatric Team (Albany, New York), 68–70
motivation: for change, and recovery from alcoholism, 136–38; for living, 20; myths about older people's, 137; for self-care, 17; for self-neglect, 94–95
myxedema, 58

National Association and State Units on Aging (NASUA), 147
National Association of Adult Protective Services Administrators (NAAPSA), 148, 149, 169
National Committee for Prevention of Elder Abuse (NCPEA), 146
National Council on Alcoholism, 128
nervous system deficits, 57
neuroendocrine system, 58
noncompliance, 14; research on, 10; and self-neglect, 9–11
nursing homes, 91; care of alcoholic in, 139; decreasing problem behavior in, 105; defining self-neglect in, 93–98; food for resident in, 101–2; in-service training for staff of, 102–3; life-time risk of placement in, 92–93; medication use in, 93; promoting self-care at admission, 100; promoting self-care for resident in, 100–5; revolving door syndrome in, 139; room choice by resident, 101; self-neglect in, 98–99; usage rates, 92–93. *See also* institutionalization
nutrition: and developmentally disabled adults, 112; and feeding problems, 59–61; and medical assessment, 57; in nursing home, 101–2; protein-calorie malnutrition, 61–63; and self-neglect, 59–63; and vitamin deficiencies, 50, 59, 61, 62
Nutritional Program for Older Americans, 59

obesity, 61
old age: definition of, 109–10; for mentally retarded, 110; and risk assessment, 156
Older Americans Act (1965), 59, 109, 148
organic mental disorder, 97
organic personality syndrome, 53

paranoid reactions, 48, 50, 60; appearance of symptoms, 50–51
pastoral visits, 104
paternalism, tensions between, and autonomy, 31
Pepper, Claude, 145
personal Autonomy in Long-Term Care Initiative, 167–68
personal care, 15
personal hygiene: and developmentally disabled, 113; in nursing home, 103–4; poor, 5, 7, 10, 13, 18;
personality, uncooperative, 10
personality disorders, 51–52; assessment of, 52–53
personal preferences, versus professional judgment, 37–38
phobic hermitage, 48
physical autonomy, 167–68
pneumonia, 60
political implications, of elder self-neglect, 171
powers of attorney, 43–44, 66, 158; durable, 44
practitioner: frustration of, 14–15; role of, in assisting elderly, 18, 21–24
practitioner-client relationship, 8–9, 14–15, 21–22, 23–24, 31
Prednisone, 56
President's Commission for the Study of Ethical Problems in Medicine and Biomedical Behavioral Research (1982), 29
primary control, definition of, 96

privacy, in nursing home, 103–4
problem behavior, decreasing, in nursing home, 105
professional judgment, versus personal preferences, 37–38
protective service programs, 43. *See also* adult protective services
protein deficiency, 61
pseudodementia, 49
pseudo-independent dependency, 52
psychiatric considerations, in self-neglect, 46–70
psychotropic drugs, 51
Public Law 98-527, 108

qualitative gerontology, 170–71

reactivity, effect of disturbances in, 57–58
Reagan administration, on elder abuse, 145
recovering alcoholics, on-going treatment of self-neglecting, 141–42
referrals, for self-neglect problems, 63–66; steps in, 154–56. *See also* assessment; intervention strategies
relocation, and translocation shock, 95–96
representative payees, 43, 157–58
research, 161–62, 168; and assessment refinement, 164–67; and autonomy, 167–68; broadening interest in self-care, 161–64; case identification as source of knowledge building, 169–70; coordination of resources, 171; on elder abuse, 4; health-oriented self-care focus, 162–64; informal care issue, 171–72; qualitative studies for knowledge building, 170–71; self-care task performance, 164; on self-neglect, 4–8; social and political implications, 171
resources, allocation of scarce, 32
retirement, and time management, 131–32
Retirement Research Foundation, 167
revolving door syndrome, 139–40
risk assessment: and age, 156; and ethics of intervention, 40–41
role models, lack of appropriate, for developmentally disabled adults, 113
roommates, in nursing home, 101

safety, and developmentally disabled, 112
salicylates, and malnutrition, 61
sanity, distinction between capacity and, 157
schizophrenia, 51, 60, 170
scurvy, 62
secondary control, definition of, 96–97
Select Committee on Aging, 92
self-care: adaptive compensation process of, 16–20; assessment of capacity for, 166; behavioral strategy for, 104; broadening interest in, 161–64; definition of, 15, 163; health-oriented focus on, 162–64; moral obligation for, 33; promoting, in nursing home, 99–105; and self-interest, 20; task performance in, 164. *See also* self-neglect
self-determination, preserving right of, 38–39
self-esteem, effect of loss on, 16
self-injury, 93, 95, 96
self-interest, 15–16
self-neglect: in caregiver, 34–35; community costs of, 35–37; concept of, 3–4; conceptual ambiguities, 8–12; definition of, 93–98, 128–29, 149–50; environmental factors contributing to, 21; ethical issues in working with, 27–45; family systems perspective of, 71–88; individual factors contributing to, 20–21; as intentional, 94–95; and mental disorders, 46–54; and motivation, 94–95; as multifaceted, 3; nature of, 11–12; nutritional aspects of, 59–63; psychiatric and biomedical considerations in, 46–70; referral and assessment for, 63–66; research on, 4–8; treating cases of, 21–24; and treatment compliance, 9–11. *See also* elder self-neglect; self-care

senile breakdown syndrome, 5
senior citizen discounts, 110
sense of self, 16; effect of loss on, 16; and independence, 18; and stereotyping, 19
sense of will, effect of loss on, 17
services: coordination of multiscore, 158–59; foundation for ongoing, 23
sex-role stereotyping, and assessment, 65–66
shared housing, 115
skills development, lack of, and self-neglecting behavior, 114
sleep deprivation, 57
sleep-disordered breathing, 56
smoking, 10, 56
social breakdown syndrome, 5–6, 168
social implications of elder self-neglect, 171
social intervention, steps in providing, 154–56
social security, 59, 109
Social Services Block Grant funds, 147–48
social status, and elder alcoholic self-neglect, 131
starvation hypokalemia, 62
stereotyping: and assessment, 65–66; of self-neglectors, 4–6, 12, 128; and sense of self, 6, 19; sex-role, 65–66
strangulation, sleep, 22
street people. *See* homelessness
stroke, 29, 42, 60
substance abuse, 51; intervention during on-going, 140–41; and self-neglect, 12, 14; symptoms of, 51. *See also* alcoholism; elder alcoholic self-neglect
suicide: in elderly, 48, 49, 95; subintentional, 95
support network, 19, 21; and alcoholism intervention, 141, 142; for homeless, 74; and referral for treatment, 64
sympathomimetics, 56
symptom, self-neglect as, 3

Tennessee Commission on Aging, 157

Tennessee Department of Human Services: data collected from surveys and record reviews, 152–53; key steps in providing social intervention, 154–56; legal aspects of intervention, 156–58; practice philosophy of adult protection services, 153–54; workers and coordination of multisource services, 158–59. *See also* adult protective services
terminal care plans, 38
thyroid function, 58
time management, and retirement, 131–32
training: for adult protective service workers, 156; for developmentally disabled adults, 114, 116–21; for nursing home staff, 102–3
tranquilizers, 48, 52
transient situational personality disturbance, 47
translocation shock, 95–96
treatment: and alcoholics, 137, 140–42; nursing home resident's control over, 102; refusal of, 38–39, 95; of self-neglect cases, 21–24; and substance abuse, 140–41
tuberculosis, 58, 61
twelve-step treatment programs, 142

United States, eligibility for end-stage renal dialysis in, 32
urinary tract sepsis, 61

visual effects, 57, 60; of diabetes, 151
vitamin deficiency, 50, 59, 61, 62
voluntary hospitalization, 67
vulnerability issues, 15, 16

water deprivation, 62–63
Wechsler Adult Intelligence Scale, 151–52
Wechsler Memory Scale, 151–52
well-being, personal sense of, 15, 20
widowhood, 132

zinc deficiency, 61

About the Contributors

Mary Bricker-Jenkins is Associate Professor of Social Work at Western Kentucky University. Her interests in public social services and feminist social work practice are represented in numerous publications. She has a special commitment to research and training in the public sector and to the collaborative development of empirically based models of practice with clients and service providers.

Cynthia Compton is a consultant in program development for individuals with developmental disabilities and has supervised supported living, residential services, parenting programs, and socialization programs. She is on the Executive Committee of the Missouri Chapter of the American Association of Mental Retardation.

Stephen J. Cutler is Professor of Sociology and the Bishop Robert F. Joyce Distinguished University Professor of Gerontology at the University of Vermont. He is coauthor of *Middle Start: An Experiment in the Educational Enrichment of Young Adolescents* and coeditor of *Major Social Issues: A Multidisciplinary View*. Currently, he is the editor of the *Journal of Gerontology: Social Sciences*.

Larry Dyer is affiliated with the University of Kansas as a clinical field instructor. He has worked with older adults who suffer abuse and neglect, developed services to prevent unnecessary institutionalization, and has provided counseling for alcohol and drug abuse inpatient and outpatient treatment programs.

Dorothy R. Fabian is a gerontologist consultant with the Geriatric Hip Fracture Program at the Hospital for Joint Diseases Orthopaedic Institute in New York. She has directed major programs in long-term care and community case management to support community living for frail elderly and is coeditor of *The Geriatric Imperative: Introduction to Gerontology and Clinical Geriatrics*.

Joan K. Hashimi is Associate Professor of Social Work at the University of Missouri–St. Louis. She is a former psychiatric social worker and an educational specialist in geriatric mental health, psychosocial stress, and emotional illness and is coauthor of *Isolated Elders*.

Allene M. Jackson is Program Coordinator of Aging Services at the St. Louis Association for Retarded Citizens and instructor in Gerontology at Lindenwood College. She has extensive experience in the field of aging, shared living programs, and older individuals with developmental disabilities and their families.

Eloise Rathbone-McCuan is the Associate Chief of Social Work Service at the Colmery-O'Neil V.A. Medical Center and Adjunct Professor of Social Welfare at the University of Kansas. She is author of numerous journal articles and text chapters, coeditor of *North American Elders* (Greenwood, 1988) and coauthor of *Isolated Elders*. She also conducts clinical and program research in social gerontology.

Richard L. Schiefelbusch is University Distinguished Professor Emeritus of Speech-Language and Hearing and Acting Director of the Gerontology Center at the University of Kansas. He is developing new geriatric rehabilitation models for the long-term care of aged and chronic mentally ill veterans.

William A. Tisdale is Professor of Medicine and Director of the Geriatrics Unit, Department of Medicine, at the University of Vermont. In the role of medical director in several nursing homes, he concentrates his consultative and academic work in the ethics of long-term care and geriatric patient self-care programs.

Raymond Vickers is Associate Professor of Geriatrics at the State University of New York Upstate Health Science Center at Binghamton, New York and Director of the New York State Veterans' Home. He teaches and writes in the area of psychogeriatrics and has developed models of interdisciplinary team outreach for high-risk urban and rural elderly.

Nancy R. Vosler is Associate Professor in the George Warren Brown School of Social Work at Washington University in St. Louis. She teaches advanced family systems intervention and administers a family therapy specialization for clinical social work students.

Marilyn C. Whalen is the Program Manager for Adult Protective Services for the State of Tennessee. She has long advocated for increased recognition and research on issues of self-neglect behaviors in adult clients and is active in several national organizations advancing the quality of practice in adult protective services.

Caroline T. Wilner is the Director of Social and Therapeutic Services at Meridian Healthcare Center at Brightwood in Baltimore. Her clinical practice expertise is in the field of the aging family, and she provides case management and clinical services to memory impaired adults and their families.

Linda Withers is Administrator of the McGuffey Health Care Center, Inc., in Gadsden, Alabama. She is a national consultant and trainer in clinical program development in long-term care facilities and participated in designing one of the pioneering models of nursing home care for cognitively impaired patients.